An Interdisciplinary Approach to Aging, Biohacking and Technology

An Interdisciplinary Approach to Aging, Biohacking and Technology focuses on a broad range of issues that cover everything from the most basic ways technology and biohacking influence people's everyday lives to concerns about equity, globalization and how we humans produce, consume and are consumed by our technologies.

This edited collection looks at the intersection between technology and aging, addressing the ways in which technology affects individuals, groups, local communities and entire populations. Contributions from a range of disciplines including sociology, philosophy, communications, medicine and religion provide interdisciplinary perspectives, addressing questions such as 'What is the impact of technology on adult bodies, our well-being and our safety?' The book explores risks such as surveillance technology, body modification and the Internet as well as issues in the aging journey such as the body and its modification; communication, privacy and surveillance; gerontechnology and aging in place.

Critically examining the journey of aging and exploring techniques such as biohacking, this book is for students studying aging and technology, including courses such as psychology, sociology, philosophy, cultural studies, health studies and gerontology. It will also be of interest to scholars who are curious about an interdisciplinary approach to age and technology.

L.F. Carver is an associate professor at Queen's University, Canada. Situated within a One Health perspective, Dr Carver's research and writing considers the impact of technology and surveillance on well-being and the way these intersect with gender, age and social determinants of health.

An Interdisciplinary Approach to Aging, Biohacking and Technology

Hacking Your Age

Edited by L.F. Carver

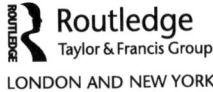

LONDON AND NEW YORK

Designed cover image: GettyImages/AndreyPopov

First published 2024
by Routledge
4 Park Square, Milton Park, Abingdon, Oxon OX14 4RN

and by Routledge
605 Third Avenue, New York, NY 10158

Routledge is an imprint of the Taylor & Francis Group, an informa business

© 2024 selection and editorial matter, L.F. Carver; individual chapters, the contributors

The right of L.F. Carver to be identified as the author of the editorial material, and of the authors for their individual chapters, has been asserted in accordance with sections 77 and 78 of the Copyright, Designs and Patents Act 1988.

British Library Cataloguing-in-Publication Data
A catalogue record for this book is available from the British Library

ISBN: 978-1-032-61727-5 (hbk)
ISBN: 978-1-032-60226-4 (pbk)
ISBN: 978-1-032-61728-2 (ebk)

DOI: 10.4324/9781032617282

Typeset in Galliard
by Apex CoVantage, LLC

Contents

Contributors

L.F. Carver, PhD, is an Associate Professor in the Faculty of Health Sciences at Queen's University, Canada as well as being the Editor-in-Chief of open access journals Aging and (Geron) Technology and One Health Innovation. Situated within a One Health perspective, Dr. Carver's research and writing is focused on the well-being of humans, non-human animals and the environment. Additionally, Dr. Carver looks at the impact of technology and surveillance on well-being and the way these intersect with gender, age and social determinants of health.

Colin Farrelly, PhD, is a professor in the Department of Political Studies (cross-appointed with philosophy) at Queen's University in Canada. He is the author of *Genetic Ethics: An Introduction* (Polity Books, 2018) and *Biologically Modified Justice* (Cambridge University Press, 2016) and journal articles in *Aging Cell, The Journals of Gerontology Series A – Biological Sciences and Medical Sciences, Rejuvenation Research, Biogerontology, Aging and Disease, Public Health Ethics, BMJ and Preventive Medicine.*

Jessica Percy-Campbell holds a PhD in political science from the University of Victoria, where she is also a sessional instructor (The Politics of Surveillance). Her research critically analyses the growing ubiquity of smart-home technology and the subsequent privacy and surveillance implications for older adults. She enjoys exploring Vancouver Island and B.C.'s lower mainland in her spare time.

Dr John Puxty, MD, is currently Associate Professor and Chair of the Division of Geriatric Medicine in the Department of Medicine at Queen's University. He is Director of the Centre for Studies in Aging and Health at Providence Care, Clinical Lead for the Southeast Specialized Geriatric Services, Integrated Memory Disorder Clinics at Providence Care Hospital and Chair of the Ontario Interdisciplinary Council for Aging and Health. He has certification as an internal medicine specialist in geriatric medicine in both Britain and Canada.

Valerie Steeves, PhD, is a Full Professor, Department of Criminology, at Ottawa University. Dr Steeves' main area of research focuses on the impact of new technologies on human rights. She is the principal investigator of The e-Quality Project, a SSHRC funded partnership of researchers, educators, advocates, civil society groups and policymakers who are interested in examining the impact of online commercial profiling. Dr Steeves has appeared as an expert witness before a number of parliamentary committees regarding privacy legislation and has worked with a number of government departments to develop privacy education curriculum and materials. Her game Privacy Playground was awarded the Bronze Medal at the 2006 Summit Creative Awards Competition, an international competition involving thousands of entries from 26 countries.

Tracy J. Trothen, PhD, is a professor of ethics at Queen's University, jointly appointed to the School of Religion and the School of Rehabilitation Therapy. Trothen is the author or editor of numerous articles, chapters and ten books, including her award-winning co-authored 2021 book *Religion and the Technological Future: An Introduction to Biohacking, A.I., and Transhumanism*. She co-chairs the American Academy of Religion's (AAR), Artificial Intelligence Seminar and is a fellow of the International Society for Science and Religion (ISSR).

Introduction

L.F. Carver

Biohacking and biotechnology are among the most interesting and intellectually challenging topics to explore in modern society. Whether you embrace or abhor technology, it is now ubiquitous, promising liberation from mundane tasks (e.g., turning on lights and unlocking doors) and even thought processes (such as remembering your schedule or your shopping lists). Biohacking takes things to a whole new level: What if you could hack aging? No wrinkles, no loss of abilities – what if you could stay "young" forever? In many ways, the pursuit of anti-aging biohacks and biotechnology is the pursuit of youth, or at least youthful life.

This book covers a broad range of issues from the most basic ways technology and biohacking influence people's everyday lives through to concerns about equity, globalization, and how we humans produce, consume, and are consumed by our technologies. None of the technologies discussed herein promise immortality. However, this book provides a corrective look at the intersection between technology and aging. It examines understandings people have taken for granted about the world around them and critically analyses the ways in which technology affects individuals, groups, local communities, and entire populations. Learning to look at techniques such as biohacking and technological tools for aging with a critical eye can be a life-altering experience.

The dive into the uses of biohacking and biotechnology is fascinating and empowering when an individual can take control of technology, rather than allowing the technology and the industrial complex behind it to control the person. But first, certain terminology and knowledge are required to understand *hacking aging*.

Frame of Reference

The terms "biohack/biohacking", "biotechnology", and "gerontechnology" are used throughout this book. These three areas have considerable overlap, so, to clarify the terms as they are used in this collection, we will briefly review them in the following.

DOI: 10.4324/9781032617282-1

Biohacking is do-it-yourself experimentation, generally with the goal of enhancing health or attributes such as sight, hearing, or mobility. Simple biohacks can include cold showers, calorie restriction, exercise, and infrared light therapy, to name a few. Biohacking may or may not include the use of biotechnology, for example, by incorporating technology into the body, such as implantable radio-frequency identification (RFID) tags that eliminate the need for passwords and open-door locks. Biohackers are people from all walks of life with any level of education, and biohacking can be done anywhere.

Biotechnology was originally used to describe innovative work that involved the use of cells, bacteria or other organisms, often in drug or vaccine development. Now, you will find the label 'biotechnology' includes technology designed to interface with human or other living tissue – for example, implants with technology built into them such as retinal or cochlear implants – as well as wearable devices (e.g., smartwatch or glucose monitors that monitor blood glucose on a continual basis). Biotechnology is a rapidly growing field and is expected to include more and more devices and techniques over time.

Gerontechnology is the intersection of gerontology (the multidisciplinary study of aging and older humans) and technology. It is defined by the International Society for Gerontechnology as "technology and environment for independent living and social participation of older persons in good health, comfort and safety". The aging and technology sector (AgeTech) is an interdisciplinary field in a constant state of flux, creating innovative solutions to age-related challenges. It is driven primarily by profit and is estimated to be worth about $900 million in 2022 (Leith, 2019).

Hacking Your Age explores what are/will be the impacts of technology on older adults, their bodies, well-being, safety, and experience of meaning and purpose. We employ intersectional,[1] social justice and equity perspectives to explore the risks to older adults from some of these technologies, such as surveillance technology, body modification, and the Internet of Things (IoT – technologies that connect and exchange data with other devices and systems).[2] The biohacks, biotechnologies, and gerontechnologies explored in the upcoming chapters may delay death via life extension (prolonging life) and/or life enhancement (improving quality of life), but they will not grant immortality.

The overall thesis of the volume is that aging is an intersectional experience that can be enhanced or threatened by biohacking, biotechnologies, and/or gerontechnologies depending on who controls them and how they are used.

The Elephant in the Room: Death

Technologies discussed in this book are intended to enhance aging, support quality of life, and extend lives beyond their current, "normal", limit. In a discussion of strategies to enhance and/or extend life, we must be willing to openly discuss death. The attitude people have towards death influences their interest in and openness to life enhancement and/or extension (Barnett &

de La Garza, 2022). People with more positive attitudes towards death (death acceptance), either because they believe in an afterlife or they see death as an end to suffering, or as an inevitable biological sequela to life, may be *uninterested* in life extension (Esnaashari & Kargar, 2018). On the other hand, those who fear death may embrace strategies that promise to alleviate or prevent suffering and delay, or even provide an escape from, death. Many religions, cultures, and worldviews seem to embrace the idea of a longer, healthier life, as long as it is obtained in ways that are consistent with their guiding ethics, which may include issues such as equity and quality of life for all (Pew Research Center, 2013).

An Overview of the Text

In the chapters following this introduction, the authors focus directly on the exploration of aging and technology beginning by *introducing and exploring* biohacking, biotechnology, and gerontechnology in Chapter 1. This chapter introduces theoretical perspectives on aging as well as opens the discussion of issues surrounding privacy and surveillance that are elaborated in later chapters. It provides examples of the ways that biohacking, biotechnology, and gerontechnology enhance the experience of aging as well as pointing out some of the pitfalls. However, it does not attempt to help with the philosophical issues associated with life enhancement, extension, and even the elusive pursuit of eternal life. That challenge is addressed in Chapter 2.

Chapter 2 is the heart of this text: the *philosophical struggles* associated with life extension and tampering with death. The perspective draws directly from philosophic study. To animate this concept, the chapter addresses the biology of aging and discusses the imperative to promote healthy aging, as well as the associated challenges. The specific thesis advanced and defended is that the aspiration to achieve healthy aging will require humanity to intervene in the way humans biologically age. It introduces theoretical paradigms that have been employed by researchers to understand the process of aging and the effects of aging, *senescence*.

Chapter 3 explores significant *ethical issues*, including what it means to be human, the importance of interdependence, and the impact of ageism as well as social justice on older adults. This chapter points out that *not everyone is treated equally and/or equitably*. It underscores that the treatment of others is influenced by intersectional factors such as racialization, gender and sexual identity, socio-economic status and ableism, among other biases, and can result in systemic power imbalances. Chapter 3 also explores the possible social implications of radical life-extending technologies. This chapter grapples with ethical perspectives on life enhancement and/or extension, including those rooted in religion. We acknowledge in advance that the subject is far more complicated than can be addressed in a single chapter.

In the second half of the book, Hacking Your Age looks at specific applications of technology.

Chapter 4 considers the ways in which technology can support *people with dementia (PwD) and their caregivers*. This chapter reviews a number of technologies and evidence for the appropriateness of use with PwD. However, it also points out that the efficacy of the technology is irrelevant if people don't use it. Although older adults, in general, are interested in and use many types of technology, they are also concerned about costs and the loss of privacy inherent in devices that reveal the location and activities of the user.

Chapter 5 focuses on *aging in a smart home*. It examines digital home assistants (DHAs) – the "brain" behind a functioning smart home. This chapter initiates a conversation about the consequences of using corporately controlled surveillance devices to provide care, especially as a replacement for a human caregiver. The chapter also explores the potential for abuse, through privacy violations by devices such as "always on" microphones and practices such as encouraging the adult children of PwD to search their parents' devices to see how they are being used or to "drop in" by remotely turning on cameras or audio to check what the user is doing. There is also the possibility of abuse by device manufacturers revealing private conversations and activities (Crist, 2019). DHAs can also be used to manipulate and defraud older adults. For example, cybercriminals can create DHA services that lure users to sites which mimic banking or other important services.

Finally, the Conclusion and Future Directions section takes a brief look at AgeTech (the intersection of digital innovation and longevity). In this chapter, the longevity economy (goods and services being marketed for use by older adults) is introduced. It also explains that AgeTech, by mitigating age-related deficits and functional challenges, could be the key to aging in place and remaining independent. Technologies such as artificial intelligence (AI) are touched upon, and readers are reminded that all AI engages in data collection which is vulnerable to leakage and exploitation. The chapter flags the profit-driven nature of AgeTech. Then, the chapter considers future directions in biohacking, biotechnology, and gerontechnology. It concludes by recommending that the AgeTech sector pivot away from marketing surveillance to caregivers (individuals and organizations) and focuses instead on the facilitation of user independence.

Notes

1 Intersectionality relates to different social categories such as race, class and gender and the way that these can combine to result in additional disadvantage or discrimination. From: www.oxfordlearnersdictionaries.com/definition/english/intersectional?q=intersectional

2 Internet of Things (IoT) refers to the connection of devices within everyday objects via the Internet, enabling them to share data. It includes items such as smart refrigerators, web-enabled teddy bears and smart home devices. From: www.oxfordlearnersdictionaries.com/definition/english/internet-of-things

References

Barnett, M. D., & De La Garza, J. D. (2022). Attitude toward death, not religious commitment mediates the relationship between political ideology and attitudes toward life extension. *Death Studies*, ahead-of-print, 1–8. https://doi.org/10.1080/07481187.2021.1944402

Crist, R. (2019). Amazon and Google are listening to your voice recordings. Here's what we know about that. *cnet.com*. www.cnet.com/how-to/amazon-and-google-are-listening-to-your-voice-recordings-heres-what-we-know/

Esnaashari, F., & Kargar, F. R. (2018). The relation between death attitude and distress: Tolerance, aggression, and anger. *Omega*, *77*(2), 154–172. https://doi.org/10.1177/0030222815593871

International Society for Gerontechnology. (2022, April 21). *About us*. www.gerontechnology.org/about.html

Leith, C. S. (2019, June 5). Active aging perceptions and attitudes. *Consumer Technology Association*. www.cta.tech/Resources/i3-Magazine/i3-Issues/2019/May-June/Active-Aging-Perceptions-and-Attitudes

Pew Research Center. (2013). Religious leaders' views on radical life extension. *Pew Research Center*. Washington, DC. www.pewforum.org/2013/08/06/religious-leaders-views-on-radical-life-extension/

1 Biohacking and Aging Technology – A Primer

L.F. Carver

Aging is *stereotypically* viewed as a period of increasing helplessness when individuals decline from being independent self-determining adults to frail and infirm "seniors" who require support and surveillance (Carver & Mackinnon, 2020). This is by no means the case. Although the majority of older Canadians have at least one illness (Butler-Jones, 2012), many people aging with illness report that their health is "good" or "very good" despite the presence of illness (Carver et al., 2018).

Feeling unwell, not necessarily illness itself, has been linked to a lack of engagement in volunteer and civic activities as well as a decrease in physical activities resulting in more time spent in passive activities such as watching TV (Venne & Hannay, 2017). Staying active is important since the majority of older adults between the ages of 65 and 79 years are independent and take care of themselves with only 10% requiring home care. However, the percentage requiring home care increases with age. For example, approximately 45% of those 85 and older need help to stay at home (Avery, 2016).

Many older adults are active and engaged in their communities. Over 40% of older adults spend time daily socializing, communicating, as well as engaging in physical activity (Venne & Hannay, 2017). About 20% of older Canadians report that they are still in the paid workforce (Arriagada, 2018). Approximately 8% of adults aged 65–74 and 10% of those over 75 years old are engaged in civic, religious, and organizational activities on a daily basis (*ibid*). Utilizing biotechnology or biohacking and/or gerontechnology to feel healthier and/or stave off negative impacts of aging could help more older adults stay active and engaged and lower healthcare costs.

EQUITY

Equity in access to technology is a huge issue. Social determinants of health, such as lower income, rural older adults, marginalized, homeless, those with lower education, and certain genders in certain cultures, may prevent access technology to with the ease experienced by more advantaged individuals and groups. For example, just over 7% (7.3%, approximately 122,000) of Indigenous people in Canada are over 65 years old (Statistics Canada, 2018b)

DOI: 10.4324/9781032617282-2

"many of whom have low income and/or are experiencing food insecurity", factors that can restrict access to technology (Statistics Canada, 2012, p. 3). It is important to acknowledge the unique needs of individuals struggling with disadvantages in any discussion of access to technology.

AGING THEORY

Ageism "is stereotyping, prejudice, and discriminatory actions or attitudes based on chronological age" (Kang & Kim, 2022, p. 1, Iversen et al., 2009). Ageism often underpins discriminatory action by individuals and/or employers and/or governments, resulting in the loss of opportunities for health care or employment. Many older adults need or want to continue working beyond the "normal" retirement age, yet, due to age norms and ageist assumptions, face challenges due to misperceptions about their ability or desire to continue as contributing members of society.

Age norms are a form of stereotyping that suggests that certain roles or behaviours are acceptable only within certain age groups. For example, sexual behaviour is often considered the territory of the young, yet many older adults continue to engage actively in sexual interactions.

Despite that most older adults continue to feel younger inside than their chronological age (Carver, 2019), many younger adults consider them to be "other", different and impossible to relate to or understand. Four social theories of aging will be discussed *briefly* to try to understand the disconnect between the younger and older generations: modernization theory of aging, social constructionism, the life course perspective, and feminist gerontology.

Modernization Theory of Aging (Cowgill & Holmes, 1972) suggests that older adults lose power and influence in society due to industrialization, which changed where and how products were manufactured, and modernization which moved societies away from multi-generational families in agrarian communities to nuclear families located in and around the new industrial complexes. As societies modernize the status of older adults declines and their knowledge is undervalued. Quite often they are regarded as lacking an understanding of "modern" technologies and priorities. Younger adults often, and incorrectly, consider older adults out of touch with the new reality.

Social Constructionists theorize that "humans construct the world through social practices" (Allen, 2005, p. 36). Social constructionism describes the way that culture and society create meaning for a variety of aspects of life. "Labels, classifications, denotations and connotations of social identity always are products of their times" (Allen, 2005 p. 37). "Young" and "old" are both socially constructed and differ depending on the culture and the period in which they occur.

Gergen and Gergen (2000) suggest that, in the West, there has been a "dark age" of aging in which older adults were socially constructed as "ugly, toothless, sexless, incontinent, senile, confused and helpless" (p. 281). Importantly, Gergen and Gergen (2000) remind us that the scientific literature about older adults has also been socially constructed and the hypotheses presented and studied are the products of deeply embedded cultural perspectives on what constitutes older age. They pointed out that, in the year 2000, "cohorts of technologically sophisticated individuals are now entering retirement" (p. 286). Now, over two decades later, even more older adults are technologically savvy. All of this technology can be operationalized as tools in personal social construction. Utilizing social media these older adults are "sharing conceptions of the self, age, and personal value . . . [and] increasingly resist the constructions of others" (Gergen & Gergen, 2000, p. 287).

The Life-Course Perspective (Alwin, 2012) theorizes that each stage of life along with the social, economic, and physical environments in which we experience them impacts the subsequent stages. According to life course theory, longevity and health are impacted not just by genetics but also by early life experiences, combined with adversity (risks) and supports (resources) (e.g., Kuh & Ben-Shlomo, 2004). This theory integrates the role of individual decisions as well as the accumulation of risks and resources, into subsequent experiences, acknowledging that age cohort and historical time, location, agency, and relationships all affect the experience of aging. The most important events in the life course tend to be "leaving the parental home, marriage, marriage dissolution by divorce or widowhood, migration, labor force entry and exit" (Willekens, 1999, p. 23), and, for most people, the majority of these events occur before the age of 65 years.

The final theory we will discuss here is *Feminist Gerontology*. Feminist gerontology has roots in a feminist framework and in the life-course perspective (Hooyman et al., 2002). Feminism is "a means to understand the advantages and disadvantages that follow gender throughout the life course, as well as the gendered nature of power and domination collectively rather than individually" (Hooyman et al., 2002, p. 5). Unlike sex, which is biologically determined, gender itself is a social construction that, like age-related roles, differs based on the culture and the time period.

In feminist gerontology, there is an acknowledgement of the gendered aspects of parenting and caregiving, as well as differences in access to education and work opportunities. In most cultures, women are more likely to be primary caregivers for younger siblings, their own children and even aging parents. The commitment to caregiving can result in leaving school at a young age and/or an inability to engage in higher education. Caregiving also influences women's availability to work outside the home. Having limited access to employment means that women have less financial resources for day-to-day expenses as well as limiting their ability to save money for later life, including limiting pension contributions. Feminist gerontology is considered a tool for change. A tool that is "truly 'effective' only when it makes life better for men and women of all races, classes, ethnicities, and ability levels across the life course" (Hooyman et al., 2002, p. 22).

Technology and Aging

We think about technology these days as computers, cell phones, and wearables (devices that are embedded in clothing, accessories, or tattooed on the skin) but this is an oversimplification. In fact, technology has a long history and has been looked differently in every era. For example, wheelchairs (which appeared sometime between the sixth and fourth centuries BCE as wheeled furniture, and more widely used in the twelfth to seventeenth centuries AD) were an early form of technology intended to provide support to those with mobility issues. In the seventeenth century, trumpet-like devices were used as hearing aids. By the 1900s, these had evolved into electronic devices which reduced in size from large desk and/or handheld units in the 1930s to small ear-mounted devices as early as the 1950s (Mills, 2011). Although current stereotypes depict older adults as slow in embracing new technology, they were in fact early adopters of much of the technology we now take for granted (e.g., early telephones, radios, televisions, and even computers).

When aging brings challenges, technology is often offered as a way to manage, even mitigate, these difficulties. Biohacking and biotechnologies provide the opportunity to modify the aging body to delay, prevent, or address age-related changes. Gerontechnology offers ways to support, assist, and/or monitor the aging individual.

Biohacking

Biohacking has been described as citizen or do-it-yourself (DIY) biological experimentation (Hastings, 2019). The term "biohacking" is broadly used to describe the interface between technology and biology – including the application of biotechnology (e.g., implanted technology) to living things, such as the aging human body (Gasper et al., 2019). However, biohacking can also be eating a reduced calorie diet in order to repair telomeres or editing genes with clustered regularly interspaced short palindromic repeat (CRISPR) technology to improve health and well-being. It is an industry, fuelled by profit, that promises things like youthful appearance, quick weight loss, improved brain function, better health, etc. Biohacking is something that almost anyone can do at home – in the kitchen, garage or even in a car (e.g., Hastings, 2019).

Diet-related biohacks such as calorie-restricted diets (CR) or intermittent fasting (ICR) are often overlooked, but in fact, there is research to back their efficacy (e.g., Broskey et al., 2019; Schubel et al., 2018). Biohacking diet through continuous calorie restriction (CCR) is the most widely recommended calorie restriction regimen for weight loss and prevention of obesity-associated diseases (Schubel et al., 2019) and has been associated with anti-aging properties (see Broskey et al., 2019). CR/CCR is actually very important since it can counter the effects of overeating combined with lower levels of physical activity which result in loss of "skeletal muscle strength, mass and quality . . . [which] leads to the development of metabolic dysfunction" (Broskey et al., 2019, p. 170). CR/CCR is effective in addressing primary and secondary aging "by attenuating the rate of living and oxidative damage (primary aging), as well as reducing adiposity (secondary aging)" (*ibid*, p. 170).

Nutrigenomics, another diet-related biohack, occurs when we manipulate what we eat to influence gene expression over time. Nutrigenomics focuses on how different macronutrients (fatty acids and proteins) and micronutrients (vitamins) impact emotion, cognition, and behaviour (Mead, 2007). Researchers studying nutrigenomics suggest that diets could, theoretically, be designed based on individual genomes (Pavlidis et al., 2015) to avoid developing a disease to which an individual is genetically predisposed. The researchers do acknowledge that non-genetic factors (e.g., sedentary lifestyle, stress) also influence health outcomes (*ibid*).

Nootropics are another example of a biohack. These are biopharmacological biohacks that attempt to address dementia and other neurodegenerative disorders. For example, MB or methylene blue (3,7-bis(dimethylamino)-phenothiazin-5-ium chloride) has neuroprotective effects in cases of traumatic brain injury (Park et al., 2018) and may be a potential method of addressing age-related brain deterioration. Naturally occurring ginkgo biloba also seems to demonstrate "neuroprotective effects in human and animals" (Garcia et al., 2017, p. s877).

Biotechnological biohacking can include gene therapy using gene editing using CRISPR. CRISPR involves the use of short, repeated DNA sequences found in the genomes of bacteria and other microorganisms (Baumann, 2017) to edit the DNA of cultured cells and embryos. It can identify specific genomic sequences and create double-stranded breaks (DBS) that can then be repaired in such a way as to change genetic expression (*ibid.*).

Gene editing to address diseases in humans is a rapidly advancing field. For example, it has been used to effectively treat "cervical cancer by targeting high-risk HPV E6 using CRISPR-Cas9 and the A AV vector" (Yoshiba et al., 2019). Researchers have also had some success in the use of gene editing to address prostate cancer (Batir et al., 2019) and breast cancer (Dekkers et al., 2019). Issues with gene editing include the fact that it can be difficult to be sure which gene to target and/or how to impact all the cells in the body when necessary (Grunewald, 2019). Currently, biohacking with CRISPR is heavily impacted by social determinants of health – as it can only be done by those with access to the funds (SES), technological know–how (education) and power (influenced by sex/gender/racialization).

Another biotechnology that can be used to biohack aging is stem cell (SC) therapy which is designed to address tissue degeneration associated with normal aging (Neves et al., 2017). Currently "bone marrow-derived allogeneic mesenchymal stem cells (MSCs) provide therapeutic benefits in heart failure patients irrespective of age" and are hypothesized to be a good candidate for the treatment of frailty (Schulman et al., 2018, p. 108). Other proposed uses for SC therapy include the treatment of Parkinson's disease, Huntington's disease, stroke, traumatic brain injury, amyotrophic lateral sclerosis, multiple sclerosis, and multiple system atrophy (Nguyen et al., 2019).

Grinders – Taking DIY Biohacking to Another Level

Grinders are members of a biohacking subculture that considers the human body hack-able. Grinders often integrate technology into their bodies to try to improve their health or function. Many grinders are also makers, using technology like 3D printing to develop the parts they need for biohacks. Makers may utilize "makerspaces" (designated spaces where makers gather to create their technologies such as the NASA Ames Research Center) or work on their own or in small unaffiliated groups.

One way that older adults can take control of the technology in their lives is to engage with the DIY world of grinders. The irony of the stereotypes that suggest that older adults are averse to technology is that it ignores the large proportion of older adults who are already engaged in a version of transhumanism – merging their bodies with technology such as pacemakers or bionic pancreas and insulin pump diabetes management technologies.

Some Issues in Biohacking

DIY biology and biohacking are not without controversy. There are concerns about ethics of genetic editing – human, animal, plant, etc. – and "entangling different views on themes such as innovation, ethics, new technologies, education, employment, and risk assessment" (Ferretti, 2019). Partially, this reflects the lack of oversight that allows biohackers to perform experiments without seeking the standard ethics reviews that limit academic researchers (e.g., controlling the ways in which animals and/or humans may be experimented on). This lack of oversight can result in a lack of quality control and standards, and an inability to ensure that experimental subjects are treated with compassion and/or the experimentation is safe and/or necessary (Dhai, 2018). Furthermore, it is possible that gene editing with CRISPR can spread rapidly throughout populations (e.g., when gene-edited animals escape or are released and interbreed with wild or feral populations) creating legal, ethical, moral, and cultural questions (Grunewald, 2019).

Vaiserman et al. (2019) point out that in biohacking for "ageing and ageing-related diseases, the effectiveness of these therapeutic options is often unsatisfactory and limited by their side-effects" (p. 100977) and that we will need a great deal of research to develop systems that can counter these challenges. Finally, the social determinants of health influence access to these methods for those who are low income or in developing countries without the medical infrastructure to support more complex forms of biohacking. However, by engaging in biohacking, many people find a way to tackle health- or aging-related issues that they otherwise would not be able to address (due to the high costs of utilizing certain techniques within the context of a corporate structure such as a hospital or medical laboratory).

Diet-based biohacking is one of the few applications of scientific research that is accessible to everyone everywhere the information is shared, irrespective of social determinants of health. But most other forms of biohacking require access to resources and/or technology.

Biotechnology

Biotechnology is the use of any technology to improve the desirable characteristics of a plant or animal, such as the amount of fruit, milk or meat produced, or to alter microorganisms (Hoyle, 2004) to biologically control pests, for example.[1] It can also involve innovations like cybernetics (e.g., cochlear implants, artificial retinas, and prosthetic limbs), nanotechnology, cell regeneration and whole brain emulation. In this chapter, we will not be discussing pharmaceutical or microbial biotechnology.

Since the 1960s, biotechnology (e.g., hip and knee joint replacement) has allowed older adults with painful chronic diseases such as osteoarthritis to regain mobility (Hooper, 2013). Replacement joints are generally made of ceramic or polyethylene material – although this technology is constantly evolving, as researchers try to combat issues such as post-operative infection and joint loosening over time (AJRR, 2014). Millions of these procedures are performed annually around the world generally in people between 58 and 68 years old, depending on the location (Hooper, 2013; AJRR, 2014; Arija et al., 2011). The demand for joint replacements is expected to increase as the world population ages (e.g., Hooper, 2013). However, since the late 1990s, patient information and information on the joint replacements have been stored in registries around the world (Hooper, 2013; AJRR, 2014; Arija et al., 2011), adding to the mass of personal health data that may be vulnerable to exploitation.

Cyborgs Among Us

In science fiction, Cyborgs are a blend of humans and machines. There are in fact a multitude of cybernetic implants already in common use (e.g., pacemakers, cochlear implants, artificial retinas, and "bionic" limbs)[2] or under development to address both disease-related issues (e.g., managing heart-related challenges or restoring sight). Cybernetic enhancements in use and/or under development include implants and integrated technology intended to address age-related challenges such as loss of limb, mobility, and strength, while others are trying to restore memory, enabling individuals to live fuller lives with memory loss.

Biotechnology is widely used to address heart problems. One of the most familiar examples of biotechnology is the pacemaker, which has been used for decades to correct an abnormal heartbeat by sending continuous or on-demand electrical impulses to the heart, thus controlling abnormal heartbeats (Aquilina, 2006). Another implanted device for heart-related issues is a cardioverter-defibrillator (ICD) which shocks the heart out of potentially fatal abnormal rhythms.

Hearing loss is another age-related problem with biotechnological solutions. It is potentially debilitating for older adults, impacting approximately 25% of older adults between the age of 65 and 74 years. Hearing loss has been associated with social isolation, depression, poor health outcomes, cognitive impairment, and increased risk of fall and hospitalization (Lin et al., 2012). However, cochlear implant (CI) biotechnology has been used effectively in older adults with moderate-to-profound hearing loss (*ibid*).

Vision loss has also been tackled by biotechnology. Devices such as the Argus II can send signals from a camera built into a pair of glasses to a cluster of electrodes implanted at the back of the eye (Servick, 2019) partially restoring vision in participants with age-related macular degeneration (AMD) (Flores et al., 2019). Unlike the bulky systems mentioned earlier, the artificial retina is "a millimeter-scale, intelligent apparatus designed as a replacement for these systems, while executing simple image processing tasks" (Berco & Ang, 2019, p. 1).

There are issues associated with implantable biotechnology. Those with a neural interface in the brain can cause scarring in the brain around implanted wires, potentially introducing infection (Ordaz et al., 2017). There is also the concern that the light source used in optogenetics (vision-related implants), while promising sharper vision, may also be in danger of overheating and causing tissue damage (*ibid*). And, of course, social determinants of health such as income and access to healthcare impact access to advanced biotechnology, especially for people with low income and/or in developing countries. As well, much of this technology will be controlled by a few large corporations who will have the power to decide who benefits, potentially limiting access by those at lower socioeconomic levels, or in certain geographic areas, widening equity gaps (Stucke, 2020).

Aesthetic Surgery – Body Modification

No discussion of the *hacking age* would be complete without considering aesthetic surgery for body modification. Body modification is defined as "procedures to achieve permanent alterations of the human body" (Stirn et al., 2011, p. 359). And, although they are forms of body modification, piercing, tattoos, and scarification will not be discussed here as they are not generally utilized as anti-aging techniques. Historically bodies were surgically modified to conform to aesthetic norms – for example, to make the female body more consistent with the beauty norms of the day. However, "as we grow older the body displays physical signs of aging, and we now have surgical procedures that aim to 'correct' the signs of ageing" (Alsop & Lennon, 2018, p. 99).

Body modification through cosmetic/aesthetic surgeries including implants, facelifts, and body sculpting is performed at high rates around the world. "Shaping implants" do not contain technology, instead, they are used to change and shape the appearance of specific body areas including buttocks, penis, chest, calf, bicep and triceps, shoulder muscle (deltoid), abdominal muscle, forearm muscle, wrist and thigh implants. Generally, these implants are made of semi-solid, rubberized silicone that can be permanently positioned without risk of absorption by, or distributed through, the body. Other methods of body modification include liposuction and fat transfer. Body modification has become a multibillion-dollar industry over the last decade. This market growth has been fuelled by the development of noninvasive options for treating fat deposits (Bonan et al., 2018), cellulite (Alizadeh et al., 2016), and microfocused ultrasound to rejuvenate skin (Kerscher et al., 2019).

According to Lane (2017), there are three key elements to body modification: such modifications are voluntary, they are aesthetic and intended to alter the appearance of the human body, and they are for non-medical purposes. The desire to use body modification to achieve a different appearance may be more than just a physical change. "Aesthetic surgery is currently located within a makeover culture, marketed and consumed as an exercise in agency, in self-making" (Alsop & Lennon, 2018, p. 101), so body modification may be a way to manifest self-identity.

Choosing to modify the body is an expression of agency when the *consumer* engages in modification to create a body that reflects how they see themselves. In the case of older adults, it may be used to bring the external appearance more in line with the internal concept of the self, bringing the body to reflect the age inside (Carver, 2019) rather than chronological age. Edmonds (2010) studied body modification in Brazil and suggested that it was a type of *psychological healing*. This is supported by other researchers who conclude that "by looking younger, more western, healthier or more sexually attractive our inter-subjective relations were improved" (Alsop & Lennon, 2018, p. 101).

Body modification has been "repositioned as something 'normal' people could have, something you didn't have to be psychologically compromised to desire" (Jones, 2008, p. 25). It is being done by women and men to combat signs of aging such as hair transplants to counter balding, breast and buttock implants and lifts to counter stretching and sagging, and liposuction for body sculpting to reflect the normative "young" body. Body modifiers are now considered "consumers rather than patients; the body that ensues is a product to be purchased" (Alsop & Lennon, 2018, p. 98). It is increasingly normalized through marketing (*ibid*).

Cosmetic surgeries including implants, facelifts, and body sculpting are commonplace procedures. Globally, breast surgery involving lifts and shaping implants brought in 1.2 billion USD in 2016. This market is expected to continue to grow due to both the desire to have reconstructive surgery after breast cancer removal and to bring bodies into line with the beauty norm of youthfulness. Body-modification techniques as a whole are not without controversy – both in terms of their safety (e.g., the toxicity of some breast and other body-shaping implants) and their intent (to make bodies conform to a socially constructed image of the ideal).

Gerontechnology

Gerontechnology is used to help older adults to age in place, by monitoring health status, supporting social connection, and providing activities for leisure time. This field of study was developed in the late 1980s, beginning with a research team at the Eindhoven University of Technology, in the Netherlands. Early gerontechnologists had the goal of enhancing the integration of engineering with traditional aging research (Graafmans, 2016). The Dutch government encouraged the development of this interdisciplinary field, bringing together people from disciplines such as health care, welfare, engineering, architecture, and industrial design to work to establish better physical environments and improve quality of life, as well as to support the independence of older adults. Now, decades later, gerontechnology has made it to the mainstream and is often referred to as AgeTech, especially in commercial markets.

In this book, the term "gerontechnology" refers to technologies applied to mitigate age-related challenges. Stereotypically, technology utilized by older adults is associated with illness and lack of capacity in some areas. However, although gerontechnological devices can be assistive technology, they can also be technologies that create inclusive environments to support independent living and social participation for older adults, whether or not they have health issues, including supporting older adults' leisure activities.

When they are used to promote social connection and/or monitor health, common devices such as smartphones, tablets, and wearables can be considered gerontechnology. For example, wearables like smartwatches can record health data 24 hours a day (Alley et al., 2016) as well as providing GPS tracking, to locate wandering dementia patients or lost joggers, and promoting social connectivity through social media notifications. However, there is a potential *downside* since smartwatches, like smartphones and tablets, can also be used for surveillance – via GPS monitoring or just by text/email/phone contact – with or without the older adult's permission (Carver & Mackinnon, 2020).

Ambient-Assisted Living (AAL)/Home-Monitoring Systems

Ambient-Assisted Living (AAL) gerontechnologies are home monitoring systems allowing for around-the-clock monitoring of older adults. AAL technology is installed as a system of sensors that record data in specific locations and then contact caregivers if the sensors indicate that the data collected is outside of "normal" range. For example, more time than usual spent in the bathroom or abnormal heart rate (Epstein et al., 2016; Berridge, 2016). Often sensors are put on doors, such as refrigerator, medicine cabinet, or bathroom, and can record when the door is opened or closed. They may also be installed on the stove to report when it is on or off (Berridge, 2016). Bedroom sensors can record respiration, heart rate, and movements while the older adult is in bed, regardless of whether they are sleeping or engaging in sexual activity. AAL systems run data through an algorithm and use a database server and web portal to store data and make it available to caregivers. AAL systems are generally more cost-effective than 24 hours a day human monitoring.

More advanced systems also exist, such as Emerald, a wall-mounted touchless sensor that analyses radio waves to track motion, social activity, and sleep pattern. Research has shown that "the Emerald device can generate outcome measures that may be more sensitive to change than traditional clinical outcome measures".

Technology and Privacy

Since gerontechnology has the ability to collect data on the physical characteristics, location and activities of older adults (Berridge, 2016), it functions as a surveillance system (Carver & Mackinnon, 2020). Although these devices are often marketed to promote independence and autonomy, it is important to ensure that access to technology is coupled with privacy protection and the prevention of abuse.

Many older adults, themselves, express privacy concerns when offered AAL systems (see Berridge, 2016; Epstein et al., 2016) and/or devices such as smartphones and wearables that can track their whereabouts and/or record their vital signs. For example, AAL systems or technology like Emerald that are always on and undetectable can mean that older adults are unaware of the extent to which their lives are under observation. There is no respite for privacy or intimacy unobserved by family and/or caregivers unless the older adult under observation knows how to shut it off to gain some privacy.

Personal Health Data

The COVID-19 pandemic has exacerbated an important issue with technological surveillance: the exploitation of personal health data (Carver & Mackinnon, 2020). The data gathered by the many devices used by or for older adults can be combined with personal health data from primary healthcare providers (such as the family doctor). Together the surveillance and personal health data can be used for purposes other than medical care or the direct protection of the user. This happens regularly when insurers combine the personal health information they obtain when an individual applies for insurance coverage with data collected by some companies as part of incentive-based "health promotion" programs (e.g., SilverSneakers[3] offered by Medicare or Manulife's Vitality).[4] Where a government chooses to permit "off label" use of this data – usages other than the intended ones – there may be privacy consequences (Bertot et al., 2014).

Consent

When health information is collected by physicians for the provision of health care, that data is guaranteed to be kept protected and confidential. Patient consent is implied to extend that information to the circle of care – the team of doctors, nurses, and other healthcare providers that care for a given individual – for the purposes of facilitating the provision of medical care to a patient/client. However, massive databases[5,6] have been built in response to COVID-19 to amalgamate information from primary-care physicians with data on individuals from hospitals, drug programs, emergency response teams, and potentially linking to consumer data from credit and points cards as well as possibly connecting COVID Alert Apps' GPS data from cell phones.

The Ontario Health Data Platform (OHDP) is an example of *off-label* data utilization (use other than the original purpose). In the OHDP, personal health data is transferred *from* the medical-care setting *to* an amalgamated mega-database where it can be accessed for purposes other than healthcare provision. The OHDP is a large health dataset that includes information currently held across various organizations, such as personal health records from family physicians or public health testing information, and integrates individuals' data "so researchers can analyse and gain insights to help with understanding and combatting COVID-19".[7] And, unfortunately, once these mega-databases are created, they are very difficult to disassemble. It is also important to note, "the public acceptability of third party access to detailed health care datasets is, at best, unclear" (Keen et al., 2013).

These off-label uses of data are problematic because people have not had the opportunity to decide if they are willing to have their health information used in these ways. And, "the right to privacy is essentially the right of individuals to have their own domain, separated from the public" (Becker, 2019, p. 308). Thus, the lack of opportunity to consent or opt-out violates the right to privacy.

Having the opportunity to decide how and when personal medical information is used and released can be important in terms of privacy and peace of mind, it is not enough to assert that privacy has been an integral part of the design of mega-databases. Allowing people to request to review their data as it appears and choose whether or not to consent to their data being included in that database and/or whether it should made available for other research and/or for commercial purposes would increase data sovereignty for older adults (Kilzi, 2021).

Anonymity

The second issue with amalgamated mega-health databases is that most data in these large health databases *has not been anonymized*. To anonymize, all identifying information would need to be removed. Instead, it has been de-identified. When data is de-identified, details such as name and street address are usually excluded from the database, but indirect identifiers such as postal/zip code, date of birth, ethnicity, sex, gender, age, income, education, diagnosis, diagnostic tests, and surgeries/treatments are still present. The more indirect identifiers included in the database, the greater the chances that an individual may be re-identified. Further, when personal health data is combined in a database with non-health data such as transactions at favourite stores or websites, apps utilized and/or social media behaviour, the opportunities for re-identification expand. For example, when multiple data points are combined such as GPS coordinates, diagnoses, income, sex, and/or ethnicity certain vulnerable individuals and groups can be identified, especially in rural areas where there may be small numbers of people in certain categories.

Privacy Protection

Privacy can be partially protected through effective legislation, and by trusted data users being trustworthy, but both are vulnerable to exploitation to serve the personal (e.g., career-building research) or organizational (e.g., monetization) needs of the users. Further, when large amounts of data are amalgamated, the mega-database can attract the attention of criminal hackers, market researchers, commercial interests, and even foreign countries. As a result, governments and organizations must proactively create policies to address privacy, security, anonymity, and consent as well as implement privacy and security measures wherever the database is housed.

Although many governments have some type of privacy protection enshrined in legislation, they can amend legislation – sometimes so quietly that very few are aware of the changes. These amendments can be used to serve new interests, sometimes for the good of citizens and other times to support a government agenda or to increase revenues by allowing commercial interests to access these unprecedentedly valuable databases. The ability to alter legislation to align with government revenue generation plans means that the government may not be a reliable protector of citizens' personal health data.

In these big data sets created by governments, alone or in cooperation with private interests, patients can't opt out because they have never opted in. The data provider has no say in how their data is used or whether it is exploited. Further, organizations can, in some circumstances, sell the data that they generate, to be utilized for scientific or market research – depending on the buyer. And, if the data governors sell the database, the patients who provided the data cannot stop the sale nor will they profit from it.

Hacking Your Age – Conclusion

Biohacking and the various forms of technology, as we have seen in this brief primer, have the potential to support older adults in the "battle" against age-related declines. Age-related challenges can certainly be hacked using the biohacks and technologies discussed earlier, including calorie restriction, plastic surgery, SC therapy, gene therapy and gene editing, cybernetics, and replacement organs, among others. However, hacking the aging body has socio-philosophical implications (Farrelly, 2024). There are also ethical implications associated with the potential for radical life extension that may be the consequence of hacking age (Trothen, 2024).

Finally, it is important to remember that there are risks associated with the use of cutting-edge technology, potentially unproven by research (in the case of biohacks and grinders). Further, there are significant risks posed by unfettered surveillance through new technologies (Carver & Mackinnon, 2020). The vulnerability of older adults can be increased when their homes are riddled with devices designed to record their every interaction, heartbeat, breath, and step. And, when governments themselves combine surveillance data with the personal health data generated through the utilization of healthcare services, the privacy risks are multiplied.

Fundamentally, biohacking and the use of biotechnology and gerontechnology can be extremely beneficial for most older adults, who use these devices for the same reasons as younger adults (e.g., for fitness goals, appointments, social connectedness, and things like heart-rate monitoring or step tracking), as well as mitigating age-related challenges. And certainly, hacking the experience of aging is exciting and provides the tantalizing image of a healthier, more active old age, and even life extension. However, equity must be considered, including the potential that biohacking, biotechnology, and gerontechnology may be limited to those with wealth and power, or sequestered in developed countries. Socially just legislation and policy must accompany anti-aging and assistive technologies, so that anyone who wants to can safely biohack aging.

Notes

1 https://nifa.usda.gov/microbial-biotechnology
2 For example, www.ossur.com/en-us/prosthetics/arms/i-limb-quantum
3 SilverSneakers.com
4 www.manulife.ca/personal/vitality.html
5 https://news.ontario.ca/en/release/56659/province-developing-new-health-data-platform-to-help-defeat-covid-19
6 www.hdrn.ca/en/public
7 https://ohdp.ca/overview/

References

AJRR. (2015). AJRR releases 2014 annual report: Hip and knee arthroplasty data for more than 200,000 procedures. *AAOS Now*, 36. https://www.aaos.org/registries/publications/ajrr-annual-report/

Alizadeh, Z., Halabchi, F., Mazaheri, R., Abolhasani, M., & Tabesh, M. (2016). Review of the mechanisms and effects of noninvasive body contouring devices on cellulite and subcutaneous fat. *International Journal of Endocrinology and Metabolism*, *14*, e36727.

Allen, B. J. (2005). Social constructionism. In *Engaging organizational communication theory and research: Multiple perspectives* (pp. 35–53). SAGE Publications, Inc.

Alley, S., Schoeppe, S., Guertler, D., Jennings, C., Duncan, M. J., & Vandelanotte, C. (2016). Interest and preferences for using advanced physical activity tracking devices: Results of a national cross-sectional survey. *BMJ Open*, *6*(7), e011243. https://doi.org/10.1136/bmjopen-2016-011243

Alsop, R., & Lennon, K. (2018). Aesthetic surgery and the expressive body. *Feminist Theory*, *19*(1), 95–112.

Alwin, D. F. (2012). Integrating varieties of life course concepts. *The Journals of Gerontology: Series B, 67B*(2), 206–220. https://doi.org/10.1093/geronb/gbr146

Aquilina, O. (2006). A brief history of cardiac pacing. *Images in Paediatric Cardiology, 8*(2), 17–81.

Arija, M. S., López Lasanta, M., Jiménez Núñez, F. G., Ureña, I., Espiño-Lorenzo, P., Romero Barco, C. M., López Belmonte, M. Á., Coret, V., Irigoyen, M. V., & Fernández Nebro, A. (2011). Annual trends in knee and hip arthroplasty in rheumatoid arthritis 1998–2007. *Reumatologia Clinica, 7*(6), 380.

Arriagada, P. (2018). A day in the life: How do older Canadians spend their time? *Insights on Canadian Society*. March. Statistics Canada Catalogue no. 75-006-X ISSN 2291-0840. https://www150.statcan.gc.ca/n1/pub/75-006-x/2018001/article/54947-eng.htm

Avery, G. (2016). *The state of seniors health care in Canada*. Canadian Medical Association. https://cma.ca/sites/default/files/2018-11/the-state-of-seniors-health-care-in-canada-september-2016.pdf

Batır, M. B., Şahin, E., & Çam, F. S. (2019). Evaluation of the CRISPR/Cas9 directed mutant TP53 gene repairing effect in human prostate cancer cell line PC-3. *Molecular Biology Reports, 46*(6), 6471–6484. https://doi.org/10.1007/s11033-019-05093-y

Baumann, K. (2017). Biotechnology: CRISPR-cas becoming more human. *Nature Reviews. Drug Discovery, 16*(9), 601.

Becker, M. (2019). Privacy in the digital age: Comparing and contrasting individual versus social approaches towards privacy. *Ethics and Information Technology, 21*(4), 307–317. https://doi.org/10.1007/s10676-019-09508-z

Berco, D., & Shenp Ang, D. (2019). Recent progress in synaptic devices paving the way toward an artificial Cogni-Retina for bionic and machine vision. *Advanced Intelligent Systems, 1*(1), 1900003. https://doi.org/10.1002/aisy.201900003

Berridge, C. (2016). Breathing room in monitored space: The impact of passive monitoring technology on privacy in independent living. *The Gerontologist, 56*(5), 807–816. https://doi.org/10.1093/geront/gnv034

Bertot, J. C., Gorham, U., Jaeger, P. T., Sarin, L. C., & Choi, H. (2014). Big data, open government and e-government: Issues, policies, and recommendations. *Information Polity, 19*(1–2), 5–16. https://doi.org/10.3233/IP-140328

Bonan, P., Marini, L., & Lotti, T. (2018). Microwaves in body sculpting: A prospective study. *Dermatologic Therapy, 32*(2), e12782. http://doi.org/10.1111/dth.12782

Broskey, N. T., Marlatt, K. L., Most, J., Erickson, M. L., Irving, B. A., & Redman, L. M. 2019). The panacea of human aging: Calorie restriction versus exercise. *Exercise and Sport Sciences Reviews, 47*(3), 169–175. https://doi.org/10.1249/JES.0000000000000193

Butler-Jones, D. (2012). Addressing the social determinants of health. *Healthcare Management Forum, 25*(3), 130–133. http://doi.org/10.1177/084047041202500303

Carver, L. F. (2019). The mask we wear: Chronological age versus subjective "age inside". *International Journal of Aging Research, 2*(29). https://doi.org/10.28933/ijoar-2019-02-2606

Carver, L. F., Beamish, R., & Phillips, S. P. (2018). Successful aging: Illness and social connections. *Geriatrics, 3*(1), 3. https://doi.org/10.3390/geriatrics3010003. www.mdpi.com/2308-3417/3/1/3

Carver, L. F., & Mackinnon, D. (2020). Health applications of gerontechnology, privacy and surveillance: A scoping review. *Surveillance and Society, 18*(2), 216–230. https://doi.org/10.24908/ss.v18i2.13240

Cowgill, D. O., & Holmes, L. D. (Eds.). (1972). *Aging and modernization*. Appleton-Century-Crofts.

Dekkers, J. F., Whittle, J. R., Vaillant, F., Chen, H., Dawson, C., Liu, K., Geurts, M. H., Herold, M. J., Clevers, H., Lindeman, G. J., & Visvader, J. E. (2019). Modeling breast cancer using CRISPR/Cas9-mediated engineering of human breast organoids. *JNCI: Journal of the National Cancer Institute, 112*(5), 540–544. https://doi.org/10.1093/jnci/djz196

Dhai, A. (2018). Advances in biotechnology: Human genome editing, artificial intelligence and the Fourth Industrial Revolution – the law and ethics should not lag behind. *South African Journal of Bioethics and Law, 11*(2), 58–59. https://doi.org/10.7196/SAJBL.2018.v11i2.00667

Edmonds, A. (2010) *Pretty modern: Beauty, sex and plastic surgery in Brazil*. Duke University Press.

Epstein, I., Aligato, A., Krimmel, T., & Mihailidis, A. (2016). Older adults' and caregivers' perspectives on in-home monitoring technology. *Journal of Gerontological Nursing, 42*(6), 43–50. https://doi.org/10.3928/00989134-20160308-02

Farrelly, C. (2024). The biology of aging and its social implications. In L.F. Carver (Ed.), *An Interdisciplinary Approach to Aging, Biohacking and Technology* (pp. 24–43). Routledge.

Ferretti, F. (2019). Mapping do-it-yourself science. *Life Sciences, Society and Policy, 15*(1), 1–23. https://doi.org/10.1186/s40504-018-0090-1

Flores, T., Huang, T., Bhuckory, M., Ho, E., Chen, Z., Dalal, R., Galambos, L., Kamins, T., Mathieson, K., & Palanker, D. (2019). Honeycomb-shaped electro-neural interface enables cellular-scale pixels in subretinal prosthesis. *Scientific Reports, 9*(1), 10657. https://doi.org/10.1038/s41598-019-47082-y

Garcia, S. H., Montes Reula, L., Portilla Fernandez, A., Pereira Sanchez, V., Olmo Lopez, N., Mancha Heredero, E., Rosero Enriquez, A. S., & Martinez Parreño, M. E. (2017). Nootropics: Emergents drugs associated with new clinical challenges. *European Psychiatry, 41*, S877–S878. https://doi.org/10.1016/j.eurpsy.2017.01.1769

Gaspar, R., Rohde, P., & Giger, J. (2019). Unconventional settings and uses of human enhancement technologies: A non-systematic review of public and experts' views on self-enhancement and DIY biology/biohacking risks. *Human Behavior and Emerging Technologies, 1*(4), 295–305. https://doi.org/10.1002/hbe2.175

Gergen, K. J., & Gergen, M. M. (2000). The new aging: Self construction and social values. In K. Warner Schaie & J. Hendricks (Eds.), *The evolution of the aging self: The societal impact on the aging process* (pp. 281–306). Springer.

Graafmans, J. A. (2016). History and incubation of gerontechnology. In S. Kwon (Ed.), *Gerontechnology: Research, practice, and principles in the field of technology and aging* (pp. 3–12). Springer. https://connect.springerpub.com/content/book/978-0-8261-2889-8/part/part01/chapter/ch01

Grunewald, S. (2019). CRISPR's creatures: Protecting wildlife in the age of genomic editing. *UCLA Journal of Environmental Law & Policy, 37*(1), 1.

Hastings, J. J. (2019). When citizens do science. *Narrative Inquiry in Bioethics, 9*(1), 33–34. https://doi.org/10.1353/nib.2019.0014

Hooper, G. (2013). The ageing population and the increasing demand for joint replacement. *New Zealand Medical Journal, 126*(1377), 5–6.

Hooyman, N., Browne, C., Ray, R., & Richardson, V. (2002). Feminist gerontology and the life course. *Gerontology & Geriatrics Education, 22*(4), 3–26

Hoyle, B. (2004). Biotechnology. In K. L. Lerner & B. W. Lerner (Eds.), *The Gale encyclopedia of science* (3rd ed., Vol. 1, pp. 540–542). Gale.

Iversen, T. N., Larsen, L., & Solem, P. E. (2009). A conceptual analysis of ageism. *Nordic Psychology, 61*(3), 4–22.

Jones, M. (2008). *Skintight: An anatomy of cosmetic surgery.* Berg.

Kang, H., & Kim, H. (2022). Ageism and psychological well-being among older adults: A systematic review. *Gerontology & Geriatric Medicine, 8,* 23337214221087023. https://doi.org/10.1177/23337214221087023

Keen, J., Calinescu, R., Paige, R., & Rooksby, J. (2013). Big data+politics=open data: The case of health care data in England. *Policy & Internet, 5,* 228–243. https://doi.org/10.1002/1944-2866.POI330

Kerscher, M., Nurrisyanti, A. T., Eiben-Nielson, C., Hartmann, S., & Lambert-Baumann, J. (2019). Skin physiology and safety of microfocused ultrasound with visualization for improving skin laxity. *Clinical, Cosmetic and Investigational Dermatology, 12,* 71–79. https://doi.org/10.2147/CCID.S188586

Kilzi, M. (2021). The anatomy of personal data sovereignty. *Forbes.* www.forbes.com/sites/forbesbusinesscouncil/2021/05/04/the-anatomy-of-personal-data-sovereignty/?sh=1e26776e61e1

Kuh, D., & Ben-Shlomo, Y. (2004). *A life course approach to chronic disease epidemiology.* Oxford University Press.

Lane, D. C. (2017). Understanding body modification: A process-based framework. *Sociology Compass, 11*(7), e12495. https://doi.org/10.1111/soc4.12495

Lin, F. R., Chien, W. W., Li, L., Clarrett, D. M., Niparko, J. K., & Francis, H. W. (2012). Cochlear implantation in older adults. *Medicine, 91*(5), 229–241. https://doi.org/10.1097/MD.0b013e31826b145a

Mead, M. N. (2007). Nutrigenomics: The genome – food interface. *Environmental Health Perspectives, 115*(12), A582–A589. https://doi.org/10.1289/ehp.115-a582

Mills, M. (2011). Hearing aids and the history of electronics miniaturization. *IEEE Annals of the History of Computing, 33*(2), 24–44. https://www.muse.jhu.edu/article/449247

Neves, J., Sousa-Victor, P., & Jasper, H. (2017). Rejuvenating strategies for stem cell-based therapies in aging. *Cell Stem Cell, 20*(2), 161–175. https://doi.org/10.1016/j.stem.2017.01.008

Nguyen, H., Zarriello, S., Coats, A., Nelson, C., Kingsbury, C., Gorsky, A., Rajani, M., Neal, E. G., & Borlongan, C. V. (2019). Stem cell therapy for neurological disorders: A focus on aging. *Neurobiology of Disease, 126,* 85–104. https://doi.org/10.1016/j.nbd.2018.09.011

Ordaz, J. D., Wu, W., & Xu, X.-M. (2017). Optogenetics and its application in neural degeneration and regeneration. *Neural Regeneration Research, 12*(8), 1197–1209. https://doi.org/10.4103/1673-5374.213532

Park, J., Choi, E., Shin, S., Lim, S., Kim, D., Baek, S., Lee, K. P., Lee, J. J., Lee, B. H., Kim, B., Jeong, K., Baik, J.-H., Kim, Y. K., & Kim, S. (2018). Nootropic nanocomplex with enhanced blood-brain barrier permeability for treatment of traumatic brain injury-associated neurodegeneration. *Journal of Controlled Release, 284,* 152–159. https://doi.org/10.1016/j.jconrel.2018.06.021

Pavlidis, C., Patrinos, G. P., & Katsila, T. (2015). Nutrigenomics: A controversy. *Applied and Translational Genomics, 4,* 50–53.

Schübel, R., Nattenmüller, J., Sookthai, D., Nonnenmacher, T., Graf, M. E., Riedl, L., Schlett, C. L., von Stackelberg, O., Johnson, T., Nabers, D., Kirsten, R., Kratz, M., Kauczor, H.-U., Ulrich, C. M., Kaaks, R., & Kühn, T. (2018). Effects of intermittent and continuous calorie restriction on body weight and metabolism over 50 wk: a randomized controlled trial. *The American Journal of Clinical Nutrition, 108*(5), 933–945. https://doi.org/10.1093/ajcn/nqy196

Schulman, I. H., Balkan, W., & Hare, J. M. (2018). Mesenchymal stem cell therapy for aging frailty. *Frontiers in Nutrition, 5,* 108. https://doi.org/10.3389/fnut.2018.00108

Servick, K. (2019, October 31). New technologies promise sharper artificial vision for blind people. *Science.* https://www.science.org/content/article/new-technologies-promise-sharper-artificial-vision-blind-people

Statistics Canada. (2012). *Aboriginal seniors in population centres in Canada* (Statistics Canada catalogue no. 89–653-X). https://www150.statcan.gc.ca/n1/pub/89-653-x/89-653-x2017013-eng.pdf

Statistics Canada. (2018b). First nations people, Métis and inuit in Canada: Diverse and growing populations. *Statistics Canada Catalogue no.89–659-X.* Statistics Canada/Statistique Canada. www150.statcan.gc.ca/n1/en/pub/89-659-x/89-659-x2018001-eng.pdf?st=KZByQhfs

Stirn, A., Oddo, S., Peregrinova, L., Philipp, S., & Hinz, A. (2011). Motivations for body piercings and tattoos – The role of sexual abuse and the frequency of body modifications. *Psychiatry Research, 190*(2–3), 359–363. https://doi.org/10.1016/j.psychres.2011.06.001

Stuke, M. (2020, April 3). *Here are all the reasons why it's a bad idea to let a few tech companies monopolize our data.* Harvard Business Review. https://hbr.org/2018/03/here-are-all-the-reasons-its-a-bad-idea-to-let-a-few-tech-companies-monopolize-our-data

Trothen, T. (2024). Anti-aging or enhancing-aging technologies? Social and religious implications of radical life extension. In L.F. Carver (Ed.), *An Interdisciplinary Approach to Aging, Biohacking and Technology* (pp. 44–62). Routledge.

Vaiserman, A., De Falco, E., Koliada, A., Maslova, O., & Balistreri, C. R. (2019). Anti-ageing gene therapy: Not so far away? *Ageing Research Reviews, 56,* 100977. doi:10.1016/j.arr.2019.100977

Venne, R., & Hannay, M. (2017). Demographics, the Third Age and partial retirement: Policy proposals to accommodate the changing picture of female retirement in Canada. *Journal of Women & Aging, 29,* 1–19. https://doi.org/10.1080/08952841.2017.1377541

Willekens, F. J. (1999). The life course: Models and analysis. In L. J. G. van Wissen & P. A. Dykstra (Eds.), *Population issues. The plenum series on demographic methods and population analysis* (pp. 23–51). Springer. https://doi.org/10.1007/978-94-011-4389-9_2

Yoshiba, T., Saga, Y., Urabe, M., Uchibori, R., Matsubara, S., Fujiwara, H., & Mizukami, H. (2019). CRISPR/Cas9-mediated cervical cancer treatment targeting human papillomavirus E6. *Oncology Letters, 17*(2), 2197–2206. https://doi.org/10.3892/ol.2018.9815

2 The Biology of Aging and Its Social Implications

Colin Farrelly

Introduction

The World Health Organization (WHO) has designated the decade 2021–2030 as the "Decade of Healthy Aging".[1] The WHO defines "healthy aging" as "the process of developing and maintaining the functional ability that enables wellbeing in older age. Functional ability is about having the capabilities that enable all people to do what they have reason to value". In a century where humanity faces so many pressing societal problems and challenges, ranging from climate change and poverty, to infectious disease and political and economic unrest, the call to promote healthy aging might strike many as a rather eccentric and trivial, or even problematic, priority. And yet the reality is that population aging, while an unprecedented success story of the mitigation of early- and mid-life mortality, also creates pressing societal challenges that humanity has never faced before in history.

This chapter will draw on insights from the biology of aging to detail why the imperative to promote healthy aging is so significant, but also so challenging. The specific thesis advanced and defended is that the aspiration to achieve healthy aging will require humanity to purposely modulate the way humans biologically age. This is the central concern of the interdisciplinary scientific field of inquiry known as "geroscience", "which strives to understand how aging enables chronic disease and seeks to develop novel multi-disease preventative and therapeutic approaches" (Kennedy et al., 2014, p. 709). To make the case that modulating aging is a socially desirable, and scientifically feasible, aspiration, attention is drawn to the following four key insights from the biology of aging:

1 Biological aging (or senescence) is not genetically programmed, and thus is the *product of evolutionary neglect*.
2 This evolutionary neglect leaves us susceptible to multi-morbidity, frailty, and disability in the *post-reproductive phase* of the lifespan.
3 Aging is *malleable* (rather than fixed).
4 Scientists are making substantive progress towards developing interventions that could slow or even reverse aging in humans.

DOI: 10.4324/9781032617282-3

Humanity possesses an *evolved* biology that was driven and shaped by evolution by natural selection. And one of the most significant consequences of this evolved biology is *aging*. Reproduction was given a higher priority than longevity, and, thus, humans are susceptible to *multi-morbidity* in the post-reproductive stage of the human lifespan.

Post-reproductive lifespans in mammals are rare (Ellis et al., 2018). A species can be characterized as having a post-reproductive stage if "a female entering the adult population can expect, on average, to live long enough to spend some of their life post-reproductive" (Ellis et al., 2018, p. 2483). Humans have a post-reproductive stage, evident by the fact that "women in modern societies can expect to live nearly one-third of their adult lives in a post-reproductive state" (Austad, 1997, p. 161). The phenomenon of population aging is a very recent development, and, as the Nobel laureate Peter Medawar (1952, p. 13) argued, more than half a century ago, *unnatural.* Historically human populations did not age as high rates of early and mid-life mortality ensured that most humans died before entering the post-reproductive phase of their lives. But over the past two hundred years, human civilizations have made significant progress in terms of reducing early-, mid-, and even late-life mortality through advances in public health (e.g., clean drinking water, immunizations, and changes in behaviour), improvements in material prosperity, birth control, medical treatments, etc. Our success in delaying disease and death, by reducing extrinsic risk factors, has created aging populations.

Life expectancy for a baby born in the world today is now age 73 and is expected to rise to age 81 by the end of this century (United Nations, 2012, p. xviii). And by the year 2050, there will be over two billion persons over the age of 60. Hence, the reason why it is important to aspire to promote healthy aging. By addressing the four key insights concerning the biology of aging, a compelling case can be made for the position that aspiring to at least slow human aging ought to be considered a major priority for public health (Butler et al., 2008; Kaeberlein et al., 2015). The aging of the human species, and its social and political implications, is not something that can be easily framed in a media sound bite or even a newspaper editorial. This stems from the fact that population aging is a complex, multifaceted phenomenon. The aging of human populations is both a success story and a story rife with pressing and complex predicaments. Aging is not only a global and universal story but also a story that is linked to issues of development, sex, and intergenerational justice. As the four key insights are detailed from the biology of aging, attention is drawn to some of the societal implications of these findings. By doing so, one can appreciate the significance, and complexity, of issues raised by the aging of human populations.

What Is Aging, and Why Do We Age?

The evolution of the aging process has long been a biological riddle, because it is difficult to explain the evolution of a trait that has apparently no benefit to the individual.

(Kowald & Kirkwood, 2016, p. 986)

In common usage, the word "aging" often refers to *chronological aging*. When someone says, "My house is 25 years old", they are referring to the duration of time, measured in human-constructed reference terms (e.g., 12 months = 1 year), the house has been in existence. *Biological aging* (or senescence) refers to something very different from chronic aging. For sexually reproducing species like humans, pigs, and horses, biological aging does not begin until after these animals have reached sexual maturity. So a child who is chronologically 12 years of age is not "biologically aging" yet. S/He will not start aging until reaching sexual maturity.

Many scholars from different disciplines (e.g., kinesiology, sociology, gerontology, and biology) study aging and thus aging itself are somewhat of a contested concept. In fact, different scholars might be referring to different things when they refer to "aging". The scientists that study the biology of aging use something like the following specific understanding of biological aging: "the progressive loss of function accompanied by decreasing fertility and increasing mortality with advancing age" (Kirkwood & Austad, 2000, p. 233). Children are *developing*, but not biologically aging and their risk of death is not advancing as they go from age 12, to age 13, and then age 14 nor is their fertility decreasing. Contrast that with the circumstances of an older adult who is currently age 80. Her/His risk of death has been increasing exponentially for over half a century. After age 80, scientists estimate the mortality risks begin to decelerate (though remain very high) and reach or closely approach a plateau after age 105 (Barbi et al., 2018).

Why does an older adult face much higher mortality and morbidity risks than a child? Simply saying "because she is much older" does not adequately answer the question. Why does getting chronologically older, after reaching sexual maturity, increase our risks of disease, frailty, disability, and death? *In The Growth of Biological Thought*, Ernst Mayr claims that no biological problem is fully solved until both the proximate and the evolutionary causation have been elucidated. And the proximate and the evolutionary causation of aging are both important to understand. Let us begin by first elaborating on the meaning of proximate and evolutionary causation, utilizing the example of a crying baby detailed by Scott-Phillips et al. (2011).

Programmed Explanations of Aging

Proximate-level explanations of phenotypes, such as a crying baby, "are concerned with the mechanisms that underpin the trait or behavior – that is, how it works" (Scott-Phillips et al., 2011, p. 38). When explaining why an infant cries, for example, a proximate level explanation will invoke the immediate causal triggers that cause infants to cry, such as separation from a caregiver, being hungry or cold. When we turn to aging itself, scientists that study the causal triggers that cause older persons to be susceptible to cancer, heart disease, dementia, and death have identified a variety of triggers that increase the risks of these problems. These include the shortening of our telomeres each time a cell divides and the oxidation of proteins, all of which diminish our body's ability to repair DNA and regulate cell proliferation.

Our immune response also decreases with age. Our bone density diminishes (making us susceptible to aches and arthritic pains). The frontal lobe and hippocampus in our brain shrink and the blood flow in the brain may decrease. Such brain alterations can make it difficult to recall names, to multi-task, etc. and increase our risk for dementia, depression, etc.

Returning now to the crying baby example, to fully understand why babies cry we must go beyond simply invoking the proximate level explanation. Telling us that babies cry because they are separated from a caregiver, or hungry or cold, does not tell us why their response is to cry versus giggling or going to sleep. The evolutionary explanation for why infants cry "appeals to the fitness benefits of the trait" (Scott-Phillips et al., 2011). Crying behaviour is adaptive, it helps improve the probability that vulnerable infants can survive the precarious stages of infancy. The infants that simply went to sleep when cold or hungry were less likely to survive and pass on their genes compared to the babies that would cry and get the attention of their caregivers. Hence, the abundance of infants that display this behaviour. Darwinian selection favours babies that are able to get their needs met over those that are less capable of doing so.

When it comes to the evolutionary explanation of aging, the story is much more complex than the story of baby behaviour. Does the aging of humans serve some evolutionary purpose or function, like crying does for infants, that is programmed and beneficial to our species? This issue is important to understand because it has significant implications for the prospect of modulating human aging.

If there is a genetic program for aging, there would be genes with the specific function to impair the functioning of the organism – that is to make it old. Under those circumstances, experiments could be designed to identify and inhibit these genes, and, hence, to modify or even abolish the aging process. However, if aging is non-programmed, the situation would be different; the search for genes that actively cause aging would be a waste of effort and it would be too easy to misinterpret the changes in gene expression that occurs with aging as primary drivers of the senescent phenotype rather than secondary responses (e.g., responses to molecular and cellular defects) (Kowald & Kirkwood, 2016, p. 987).

The idea that aging is a programmed trait that is beneficial to the species has intuitive appeal. It was first proposed over a century ago by August Weissmann (1891), who argued:

> To put it briefly, I consider that duration of life is really dependant upon adaptation to external conditions, that its length, whether longer or shorter, is governed by the needs of the species, and that it is determined by precisely the same mechanical process of regulation as that by which the structure and functions of an organism are adapted to its environment.
>
> (Weissmann, 1891, p. 9)

The idea that organismal aging, and even death, are adaptive programs is still argued for by some (Singer, 2016) more than a century after Weismann first made this conjecture. There is certainly some intuitive plausibility to the idea that, in a world with finite resources, a species might evolve the adaptations of aging and death to ensure new generations of the species can survive and have access to resources. But the intuitive traction behind this idea becomes suspect when one notes that, first, historically very few humans lived long enough to suffer age-related morbidity and mortality, and second, the alleged genetic adaptative programs must in fact be for the most common cause of death among older persons – chronic disease – since people do not die from "aging" per se. In 1951, all state and federal agencies in the United States were required to adopt a standard list of contributing and underlying causes of death. Since then, no one in the United States has died from "old age" (Hayflick, 2003). Most people who die in late life die from chronic diseases like cancer, heart disease, stroke, or Alzheimer's disease. It seems implausible to suggest that these prevalent chronic diseases were selected as a "group-level" adaptation to keep population size down in our evolutionary past when very few humans would have even lived long enough to develop such diseases.

Kirkwood and Melov (2011) explain why the programmed theory of aging is flawed: If aging truly served as a general mechanism for population control, there should be ample opportunity to see this mechanism in action, for example, senescence should be an obvious and widespread killer. The fact that senescence-associated increases in age-related mortality are far from ubiquitous, and that, even where they are observed, they contribute only to a relatively small fraction of deaths within the population, seriously undermines the argument (Kirkwood & Melov, 2011, p. R702).

In their extensive critical examination of computational models and mathematical equations for programmed aging, Kirkwood and Kowalt conclude that none withstand scrutiny.

Nonprogrammed Explanations of Aging

The tendency to view aging, death, or disease as adaptations is addressed by Randolph Nesse in his book *Good Reasons for Bad Feelings: Insights from the Frontier of Evolutionary Psychiatry*, where Nesse details how prominent this mistaken view is. When Nesse and George Williams (1996) began working together on evolutionary medicine, they tried to find an evolutionary explanation for disease. Nesse notes that this was a mistake, what he calls viewing diseases as adaptations (VDAA). Diseases are not adaptations, as the diseases themselves were not selected for by evolution. Rather, "aspects of the body that make us vulnerable to diseases do have evolutionary explanations" (Nesse, 2019, p. 14). It is this insight that explains the dominant evolutionary account of aging in the field of biogerontology – the *disposable soma theory*.

Among biologists of aging, *non-programmed* theories of aging reign supreme. Such accounts emphasize individual-level developmental adaptations, as opposed to group-level, and the trade-offs of such adaptations. The most prominent of such accounts is the *disposable soma theory* (Kirkwood, 1977;

Kirkwood & Holliday, 1979). This account of aging maintains that biological aging occurs because natural selection favours a strategy in which reproduction is made a higher biological priority (in terms of the utilization of resources) than the somatic maintenance needed for indefinite survival.

Unlike the evolutionary explanation of why babies cry (e.g., to get the attention of their caregivers to comfort, feed and warm them), the disposable soma theory explains why, in a hostile world, reproduction is prioritized over longevity. Bruce Carnes (2007) usefully describes the disposable soma account of aging as follows:

> The world is a dangerous place. Death is, for all living things on this planet, inevitable. In order for any species' existence to persist over time a solution to death must be found. And that solution, for us and for other sexually reproducing species, is reproduction. There is thus a real race between reproduction and death, and all the species alive today are, at least for the moment, winning this race. But for all the species that are now extinct, like the Mammoth and Neanderthal, the race was lost.

In *The Long Tomorrow*, Michael Rose (2005) explains how the priority of development over longevity leaves us vulnerable to health problems in the post-reproductive stage of the lifespan:

> Natural selection discards bad genes, genes like those that cause fatal childhood progeria. Bad genes cause these effects by producing inborn errors of metabolism: letting toxins accumulate, impairing brain function, and so on. Many of the diseases that kill infants are the products of such bad genes . . . Natural selection keeps genes with such devastating early effects rare, because the afflicted individuals die before reproducing. Bad genes destroy themselves when they kill the young. . . . But at later ages, the force of natural selection becomes weak. It leaves genes with late bad effects alone, because natural selection has stopped working. Its force has fallen toward zero. Bad genes that only have late effects will not be removed by natural selection. They can accumulate. There is no more automatic Darwinian screening.
>
> (Rose, 2005, p. 42)

In short, the disposable soma account of aging maintains that aging is the product of *evolutionary neglect*. In the following section, we will consider some of the health and economic consequences of this fact for the world's aging populations.

Multi-Morbidity

Historically, human life has been, as Thomas Hobbes so eloquently put it in the seventeenth century, "nasty, brutish and short". Death in the Hobbesian "state of nature" – our predicament before the creation of governments, the rule of law and any public health measures – was dominated by poverty, violence, and infectious disease. There was no "population aging" in the real or Hobbesian state of nature.

An estimated 1415 species of infectious organisms have been identified as causing disease in humans, which include 217 viruses and prions, 538 bacteria and rickettsia, 307 fungi, 66 protozoa, and 287 helminths (Taylor et al., 2001). Smallpox was the scourge of the twentieth century, as "some estimates put the death toll caused by smallpox in the twentieth century alone at 500 million people" (Koplow, 2003, p. 1). Pathogens are arguably the strongest selective pressure to drive the evolution of modern humans (Karlsson et al., 2014, p. 390).

In addition to viruses, humans are also vulnerable to hundreds of bacteria. Many bacteria cause *water-borne diseases*, such as cholera, *Escherichia coli* and dysentery. Water-borne diseases, like other infectious diseases, are a much more significant problem for developing countries that still face challenges like providing clean drinking water and sanitation. An estimated 2.4 billion people still lack improved sanitation facilities and 663 million lack improved drinking water sources. Around 946 million people practice open defecation (Unicef, 2022). Thus, poverty and a lack of resources and technology are major contributing factors to the risk of infectious disease even today.

The early- and mid-life mortality risks our species have faced in the past have shaped our biology today. Evolution by natural selection occurs for a population when there is (1) *a variation in a trait* (e.g., height, resistance to local pathogens, length of a beak, aggression, etc.), (2) *differential reproduction* (e.g., some individuals have greater reproductive success than others), and (3) *heredity* (e.g., genes that influence height, immunity, a long beak, aggression, etc.). Over time advantageous traits become more common. In our evolutionary history, which was rife with early- and mid-life morbidities and mortalities, the genes advantageous to reproductive success were passed on with greater success than those genes that reduce reproductive success (e.g., those that cause early mortality or low fertility). This point is effectively illustrated by the rarity of progeria, the disease of accelerated aging. Progeria only occurs in approximately 1 per 8 million births (NIH, 2022). And the average age of death for children with this condition is 14 years. Because progeria kills the children born with this condition before they reach sexual maturity, the genes contributing to the development of the condition are not passed on. As Rose (2005) noted, the genes that contribute to early mortality are weeded out by Darwinian screening, and thus are very rare.

The story of the genes that influence our susceptibility to chronic diseases in late life, like cancer, heart disease, stroke or AD, is very different. The force of evolution by natural selection declines after the age of reproduction. Genes that contributed to cancer in our 1970s and older, for example, did not compromise reproductive fitness in a world where humans rarely lived beyond age 50. In their extensive cross-cultural examination of longevity in hunter–gatherers, Gurven and Kaplan conclude that "human bodies are designed to function well for about seven decades in the environment in which our species evolved" (2007, p. 322). This means that a child born in the world today can expect to survive beyond the natural lifespan that evolved from our Darwinian past. This has extremely significant consequences for the health prospects of today's aging populations, especially for the aspiration to promote health (versus simply delaying death) in late life.

While, in our past, the history of humanity was the history of a world dominated by infectious disease, the world of the twenty-first century is a world dominated by chronic disease (interspersed with the sporadic worldwide outbreak of viruses). In the decade from 2005 to 2015, the World Health Organization estimates approximately 76 million people died from chronic illness in high-income countries.[2] Many people assume that chronic diseases are a problem only for the world's richest countries, when in fact the opposite is true. The number of deaths from chronic disease is even higher in the most populous countries, like China and India. It is estimated that in that same 10-year period, chronic illness caused 144 million deaths in these countries.[3] "As risk of death from infectious and parasitic diseases diminish, the degenerative diseases associated with aging, such as heart disease, stroke and cancer, become much more important" (Olshansky et al., 1993, p. 47).

Chronic diseases are complex. We cannot identify just one factor, such as smoking, pollution, a particular genetic mutation, climate change, diet or lifestyle as the sole cause of diseases like cancer, heart disease, and stroke. But what is self-evidently clear when attention is given to global morbidity and mortality data in the world today is that the risks of disease and death increase dramatically as populations age and start reaching life expectancies near the upper limits of the average human lifespan.

Lifespan Versus Healthspan

Jeffrey Fries (2005) explains how estimates of the human lifespan are arrived at:

> There are several methods of estimating the human life span. One may use the anthropological formulas, reconstruct an ideal survival curve from the tail of the present curve using the assumption that these individuals have been essentially free of disease, make extrapolations from the rectangularizing survival curve, or use estimates based on observed decline in organ reserve. All suggest an average life span of approximately 85 years, with a distribution which includes 99 percent of individuals between the ages of 70 and 100.
>
> (Fries, 2005, p. 808)

If the biology humans have today has evolved from a historical context where most humans died before what we now consider "middle age", what does this mean for the world's aging populations in terms of their health prospects as they survive beyond the ages of reproduction? This aspect of the story of global aging is one rife with human suffering and rising healthcare expenditures.

Multiple chronic conditions are evident in 62% of Americans over age 65 (Vogeli et al., 2007). The reality of *multi-morbidity* means that any significant medical breakthrough in treating any specific disease of aging is likely to have a small impact on actually increasing the number of healthy years a population can expect to live. In the year 2018, approximately 9.6 million people died of cancer worldwide.[4] Eliminating all types of cancer, for example, would be a Herculean achievement considering there are over 200 different types of cancer. And yet such a revolutionary advancement in medicine is estimated to only increase life expectancy at birth in the United States by 3.17 years for females and 3.2 years for males (Olshansky et al., 1990). Why is the number so low? Because most people who die of cancer die in late life, over age 70, and as such they are vulnerable to other chronic diseases. Eliminating all cancers would not reduce the risks of heart disease, stroke, Alzheimer's disease, etc. Any one of these chronic conditions could replace cancer as the cause of death for the majority of people who would have died from cancer.

Because humans are now living beyond the "biological warranty period" (Carnes et al., 2003) of seven decades of life, we face the daunting and expensive prospect of spending enormous amounts of money tackling each specific disease of aging to extend the period of time humans can survive by managing multi-morbidity. "Further life extension in an aging world will expose the saved population to an elevated risk for all other aging-related diseases" (Olshansky, 2018, p. 1323). Jay Olshansky (2018), a prominent advocate of supporting age retardation as a form of preventative medicine, urges that the principal outcome, and most important metric of success for medicine in an aging world, should be the extension of *healthspan* (not life extension). Aspiring to promote healthy aging by directly intervening in the aging process itself could help delay, and possibly compress, chronic disease. And the longest-lived humans provide important insight into what may be possible.

Exceptional Healthy Aging

How long can humans live? And more importantly, how long can we remain healthy? Jeanne Louise Calment, from France, died in 1997 at the age of 122. She was the oldest person whose age has been verified by official documents. What was her secret? Was she an Olympic athlete? No. Did she consume a special, healthy diet? No. Healthy aging is of course a complex phenotype, and as such both environment and genes are important. But in the case of the exceptionally long-lived (age ≥ 100) persons, like Jeanne Louise Calment, genetics is extremely important. Having a centenarian sibling increases one's chances of survival to very old age (Perls et al., 1998). Furthermore, the offspring of long-lived parents have a significantly lower prevalence of hypertension (by 23%), diabetes mellitus (by 50%), heart attacks (by 60%), and strokes (no events reported) than several age-matched control groups (Atzmon et al., 2004).

The maximum human lifespan is believed to be around 125 years (Weon & Je, 2009). The prevalence of supercentenarians (age ≥ 110), and even centenarians (age ≥ 100), is very low. In the United States and other industrialized nations, centenarians occur at a prevalence rate of about 1 per 6,000. And supercentenarians occur at a rate of about 1 per 7 million.[5] These long-lived humans are an important biological puzzle to examine not simply because they live so long, but because they typically experience a delay, and compression, of morbidity. With centenarians, for example, there are three different categories of centenarians – "delayers", "survivors", and "escapers" (Evert et al., 2003). The "delayers" are people who make it to 100 years with a delay of the onset of a common age-associated illness. For "survivors", these are people who were diagnosed with an illness prior to age 80 but survived for at least two more decades. And the third category of centenarians are "escapers", people who escaped the most lethal diseases, such as heart disease, non-skin cancer and stroke.

These exceptionally long-lived humans offer hope to researchers that we might be able to extend the average human *healthspan*, and compress the period of disease, frailty and disability at the end of life for the average person. Insights into the biology of aging reveal that the rate of biological aging is malleable and influenced by a trade-off between reproduction and longevity. The disposal soma theory predicts that a greater investment in longevity should come at a cost to reproductive fitness, and a series of studies support that conjecture. This will be our focus in the following section, as the author will review some of the findings concerning how aging can be modulated.

Modulating the Rate of Aging

The third insight from the biology of aging emphasized in this chapter is the fact that the rate of aging is *malleable* rather than fixed. A variety of experimental findings have demonstrated this is the case.

Caloric restriction (CR) has been studied for decades in a variety of species (like mice) and extends lifespan by altering the rate of biological aging. CR induces stress response pathways in organisms, which results in longer life by slowing the rate of molecular and cellular decline. What makes CR so significant is that it does not simply delay death. Longer life is not necessarily desirable if it is acquired by extending the period of time a species lives with disease, frailty, and disability. But CR actually does the opposite of this. It extends life by keeping an organism *healthy* for a longer period of time (extending the *healthspan*). Since the 1930s, scientists have known "that rats and mice that are given about 40 percent less food than they would eat on their own live about 40 percent longer than do fully fed controls" (Miller, 2002, p. 160). CR in rodents delays many of the chronic conditions associated with aging and thus can be considered an "anti-aging" intervention.

In addition to CR, castration is another intervention that has demonstrated that it is possible to alter the rate of senescence. Studies on this phenomenon reveal what the disposable soma theory of aging predicts – that there is a longevity versus reproduction trade-off. Pacific Salmon, for example, die after spawning. But if castrated, these fish can survive for years longer than intact salmon. Castrated men residing in a mental hospital lived 14 years longer than intact men in the same hospital (Hamilton & Mestler, 1969). And historical Korean eunuchs had an incidence rate of centenarians at least 130 times higher than that of present-day developed countries (Min et al., 2012).

The longevity/reproduction trade-off is even evident in less dramatic examples than castration. For example, one study compared the fertility rates of men and women with exceptional longevity (Tabatabaie et al., 2011). These individuals were young adults in the 1920s, before reliable methods of birth control were widely available. The study found that the exceptionally long lived (both males and females) had an average of 2.01 children versus 2.53 children for the control group. These differences in fertility were not related to sex or to education level. But there were developmental differences among the individuals with exceptional longevity. They tended to reach menarche a year later than average, have their first child three years later, and their last child 2.5 years later than average.

CR (let alone castration!) is too burdensome an intervention to be pursued as a gerontological intervention for human populations, but the prospect of developing a drug that mimics the effects of calorie restriction might be a viable way to safely and effectively retard aging. This brings us to the fourth and final point concerning the biology of aging: scientists may be close to developing an applied gerontological intervention.

An "Anti-Aging" Drug?

Potential drug interventions are now being extensively studied to see if they alter biological aging. Rapamycin, for example, is a drug that was developed from soil on Easter Island. It is currently used as a drug to help prevent the rejection of transplanted organs for patients undergoing organ transplants. Recent experiments, however, have found that consuming rapamycin can extend lifespan, including in mammals. Perhaps the most significant study was published in *Nature* in 2009 (Harrison et al., 2009). In that study, mice that were already 600 days old (which is roughly equivalent to a 60-year-old human) were fed rapamycin. This intervention increased the median and maximal lifespan of both male and female mice.

This novel strategy of preventative medicine, that targets the largest risk factor for chronic disease (e.g., aging), is already underway in humans with the launch of Targeting Aging with Metformin (TAME) (Barzilai et al., 2016). TAME is a clinical trial to test the drug metformin as a safe and effective intervention against several age-related diseases. Metformin has been safely utilized as a pharmacological intervention to help control type 2 diabetes for decades.

Metformin exerts its therapeutic effects, through a number of mechanisms and physiological pathways that resemble those generated by caloric restriction (CR), an experimental model known to extend life span and health span in various organisms.

(Novelle et al., 2016, p. 2)

In experiments on animals, metformin has been shown to slow aging. And now researchers are hoping for a similar effect that can be shown in humans. "If TAME demonstrates that metformin modulates aging and its diseases, beyond an isolated impact on diabetes, it would pave the way for development of next-generation drugs that directly target the biology of aging" (Barzilai et al., 2016, p. 1060).

The researchers undertaking TAME describe the significance of the study as follows:

In the TAME study, we plan to enroll 3,000 subjects, ages 65–79, in ~14 centers across the U.S. Rather than study the effects of metformin on each separate condition, we will measure time to a new occurrence of a composite outcome that includes cardiovascular events, cancer, dementia, and mortality. TAME will also assess important functional and geriatric end points.

If successful, TAME will mark a paradigm shift, moving from treating each medical condition to targeting aging per se. We expect this to facilitate the development of even better pharmacologic approaches that will ultimately reduce healthcare costs related to aging.

(Barzilai et al., 2016, p. 1063)

Altering our biology of aging to help protect against chronic disease via a drug that mimics CR might constitute one of the most significant advances in public health in this century. Robin Holliday (1932–2014) was one of the first scientists to apply modern molecular medicine to the study of aging, and he had the following to say about aging 20 years ago in the journal *The Lancet*:

At the end of this century there is still a strong emphasis on the treatment of age-associated disease, rather than on its prevention. The possibility of prevention depends on research on ageing itself. . . . Development of preventative measures will certainly lower the costs of health-care for the aged. The overall aim should not be to increase the lifespan, but to increase the healthspan. This approach will not only improve the quality of life for the elderly, but also reduce the costs of medical treatment, and diminish the burden of the very large number of people who at present care for the elderly and infirm.

(Holliday, 1999, p. SIV4)

In addition to the progress being made with potentially slowing human aging, there is some reason to be optimistic that it may, in time, be possible to actually *reverse* human aging.[6] Reversing aging is very distinct from slowing aging. And, until very recently, would have been considered more science fiction than a feasible scientific goal. But in 2015, a small clinical trial (Fahy et al., 2019) began to test if growth hormone could restore tissue in the thymus gland (behind the sternum and between the lungs). For one year, the nine participants took growth hormone in conjunction with two common diabetic medications. Researchers were surprised when they discovered, by measuring the participant's "epigenetic clock", that a year of taking these three medications did more than just slow aging, it actually *reversed* biological aging by approximately 2.5 years. The study was not designed to test reversing human aging, but it might be the catalyst needed to make that aspiration a reality one day.

The Social Significance of Global Aging

The aging of human populations, while an incredible achievement, also creates predicaments that our societies have never faced before. Living into advanced ages means that older persons are susceptible to multi-morbidity, frailty, and disability. This increases the costs of healthcare expenditures. In developing countries that do not have the wealth to fund the pensions and healthcare programs of richer countries, families must rely on remaining healthy and capable of working to make ends meet. In *The Brasilia Declaration on Ageing* (July 1996), global aging is described as a development issue, stating that healthy, older persons are a resource for their families, their communities, and the economy. Their usually unpaid and unsung contributions are indispensable for development. According to the WHO (1997):

> Aging is universal, affects every individual and family, community, and society. The numbers of older persons are growing steadily. There are gender implications: older women are disproportionately represented among the oldest old and the most disadvantaged and they constitute the backbone of caregiving.
>
> (WHO, 1997, p. 177)

The gender component of global aging adds an important *intersectional* lens to the analysis of population aging. Biological aging does not affect men and women in identical ways, just as it has differential effects on the populations of rich and poor countries. Women have longer lifespans than men. "Historically, women have lived longer than men in almost every country in the world" (Austad, 2006, p. 79). Despite their longer lifespans, women tend to have longer periods of frailty and disability, the so-called "male–female health-survival paradox" (Le Couteur et al., 2018, p. 139). Living longer with frailty in later life means women face significant health and economic challenges in late life. Promoting healthy aging via an aging intervention could help ameliorate many of these vulnerabilities.

Furthermore, as the WHO statement makes clear, the caring (typically unpaid) duties for older parents typically fall to female family members. Keeping older persons healthier for longer, and compressing the period of disease and frailty at the end of life, could help mitigate (rather than exacerbate) these unequal (gendered) caring duties (Farrelly, 2023a).

One common response to the call for modulating human aging via a drug that mimics caloric restriction, or that activates the longevity genes already active in the longest-lived humans, is to argue we should simply pursue lifestyle modifications versus drug development to promote health in late life. This response posits a false dichotomy, implying that exercise would confer similar health benefits to CR and other aging interventions. This is not substantiated by experimental results. Exercise certainly does have health dividends for older persons.

> Moderate and high physical activity levels have been demonstrated to lead to 1.3 and 3.7 years more in total life expectancy and 1.1 and 3.2 more years lived without cardiovascular disease, respectively, for men aged 50 years or older compared with those who maintained a low physical activity level. For women the differences were 1.5 and 3.5 years in total life expectancy and 1.3 and 3.3 more years lived free of cardiovascular disease, respectively.
>
> (Franco et al., 2005, p. 2355)

Exercise can increase life expectancy by altering the effects of what Holloszy and Fontana (2007) call "secondary aging", but that has a much smaller impact than altering "primary aging". Secondary aging is the "deterioration in tissue structure and biological function that is secondary to disease processes and harmful environmental factors" (Holloszy & Fontana, 2007, p. 709). Aspiring to achieve healthy aging should of course take seriously the goals of encouraging healthy diets and lifestyles, and better work/leisure balance and city designs that permit humans to connect with nature and be physically active. However, exercise does not alter "primary aging" (defined as "physiological declines attributable to the aging process itself", Racette et al., 2006, p. 949). Unlike exercise, caloric restriction does alter primary aging. "CR mitigates central mechanisms involved in primary aging in both short-term and long-term trials by reducing energy flux and oxidative stress, as well as improving mitochondrial function" (Broskey et al., 2019, p. 170). An applied gerontological intervention that alters the inborn aging process could increase the human healthspan and compress the time we survive with multi-morbidity and frailty. This would lead to significant health and economic benefits.

"About 96% of infants born in developed nations today will live to age 50 years or older, more than 84% will survive to age 65 years or older, and 75% to 77% of all deaths will predictably occur between age 65 and 95 years" (Olshansky, 2018, p. 1323). Developing countries are still lagging behind developed countries in this respect. However, most people born in the world today can expect to live long enough to become a senior and will most likely die from one of the chronic diseases of aging. This shift from the historical norm, where most death and disease occurred early in life, to the predicament today, where most disease occurs in late life, amplifies the importance of aspiring to promote healthy aging. Aging populations are vulnerable to chronic disease and disability because the force of evolution by natural selection declines in late life. This means that genes that cause deleterious mutations that lead to cancer, heart disease and stroke after age 70 are passed on without being weeded out by Darwinian selection.

Raising the prospect of altering human aging provokes many different emotive responses, many of which are oppositional to talk of increasing the human lifespan rather than healthspan. Sometimes these opposition sentiments are predicated on pure ageism, and thus the critic does not see the value of adding more life to the years of older persons because they place a lower value on an older person's life. Robert Butler, the first director of the NIH's National Institutes of Aging, coined the term "ageism" in 1969, a term which means the systematic stereotyping of, and discrimination against, people because they are old. Ageism is reflected in such colloquialisms for elders as "coot", "croon", "geezer", "hag", . . . "out to pasture", "over the hill", and "washed up" (Palmore, 1999). So, those advocating for healthy aging are likely to encounter ageist attitudes.

Second, opposition to talk of increasing the human lifespan is sometimes predicated on the false belief that health is a *zero-sum game*. A zero-sum game is a situation where improvements to one person or group of people entail a diminishment in the wellbeing to others. That increases in health to some people must come at a cost to the health of others. But this is false. The amount of health available to the world's aging populations is not fixed. Nor do improvements in health and life expectancy create (all-things-considered) social ills. Typically, a healthy population is a crucial factor in helping a society remain economically viable over time. This does not mean that there might not be societal consequences worth seriously considering if we extend the human healthspan, such as the impact on how long we expect people to work, or the impact on population growth and climate change. But the appropriate response to any such concerns is to address those problems directly versus forfeiting the health benefits of an applied gerontological intervention. Furthermore, healthy aging can help protect older populations from some of the risks posed by global warming (Farrelly, 2023b). Older persons are more vulnerable to extreme weather events and infectious diseases. An applied aging intervention that helps improve our immune system and general health in late life ought to be considered a vital element of an *adaptation* response to the realities of global warming.

And third, there is the legitimate concern about *equitable access* to any prospective aging intervention. Will it only be available to those living in rich developed countries versus people living in developing countries? This is a legitimate concern, but not an *objection*[7] to developing an aging intervention. The WHO aspiration to promote healthy aging is a *global* aspiration. If we assume that humans have a right to health, including health in late life, this right does not diminish (let alone extinguish) simply because of one's chronological age. A commitment to modulating human aging should be a global aspiration, and thus the fair diffusion of an applied gerontological intervention ought to be taken seriously.

One way of assessing this worry is to draw attention to the different diffusion challenges which face medical, and other, technological advances. The benefits of sanitation, for example, are unequally accessible to the global population. However, saying this does not entail that we have compelling grounds for *forfeiting* the benefits of the sanitation revolution. The goal ought to be to ensure everyone enjoys access to improved sanitation. Why aren't the benefits of the sanitation revolution equally accessible? The reasons why health innovations are not equally accessible to all are varied and complex, and often dependent on the type of intervention in question. For example, the obstacles to universalising the benefits of smoke cessation, for example, are very different from the obstacles that arise with sanitation, immunizations, chemotherapy, and triple bypass heart surgery.

An intervention that slows down aging via consuming a diabetic drug like metformin would not face the same kind of accessibility challenges that face sanitation, chemotherapy, or heart surgery. Metformin has already been available for decades and has a good safety record. As a generic drug, it is not prohibitively expensive.

Once an applied gerontological intervention in drug form has been developed and tested for safety and efficacy, its wide dispersion should be relatively straightforward. The obstacles to diffusing such a pill are arguably comparable to those facing the provision of micronutrient supplements (to combat vitamin A and iron deficiencies, for example) or the birth control pill than to sanitation or major surgery. So, there are good reasons for being optimistic that an aging intervention would be more accessible to the world's poor than the expensive medical interventions which often just help us manage disease in late life.

Conclusion

Recall, from the introduction, that the WHO describes healthy aging as "the process of developing and maintaining the functional ability that enables wellbeing in older age. Functional ability is about having the capabilities that enable all people to do what they have reason to value". Many different factors influence our opportunities for wellbeing over the human lifespan – the culture we live in, our affluence, the environment, the social security, healthcare provided (or absent) in our society, etc.

The focus of this chapter has been on just one significant factor that impacts our wellbeing – *senescence* itself. This was done for two reasons. First, outside of the field of geroscience, very little attention is given to the biology of aging and how it makes us susceptible to a host of diseases and disabilities. Second, over the past two decades, amazing advances have been made that make the prospect of an applied gerontological intervention really a question of *when* it will be developed versus *if* it will ever be developed. And, with a projected 2+ billion people expected to be living over the age of 60 by the year 2050, the time is ripe for addressing the aspirations of healthy aging.

Our evolved biology prioritizes reproductive fitness over longevity. And a consequence of this trade-off is that as humans live into the post-reproductive phase of the lifespan, we are susceptible to multi-morbidity. If we do not alter human aging itself, the goal of achieving healthy aging will be significantly compromised and limited. As we keep people alive longer by managing multi-morbidity with a cocktail of daily prescriptions, we run the risk of simply extending the period of time we can stave off death versus actually improving our *quality of life* in late life. And what really counts, in the end, is adding life to years versus years to life. Hence, why any applied gerontological intervention would have such profound significance for the world's aging populations this century.

Notes

1 See www.who.int/ageing/decade-of-healthy-ageing?fbclid=IwAR3zSt7tIm4WQx7 MARegSaKdqNRzJS3Ka3IqP0kJolnSutF-0Adqt3mEfww
2 www.who.int/chp/chronic_disease_report/media/hi_income.pdf
3 www.who.int/chp/chronic_disease_report/media/lower_middle.pdf
4 www.who.int/news-room/fact-sheets/detail/cancer
5 Boston University's New England Centenarian Study at: www.bumc.bu.edu/ centenarian/overview
6 See www.nature.com/articles/d41586-019-02638-w
   In *Beyond Humanity*, Allen Buchanan makes a useful distinction between a *concern* about biomedical enhancement, and *an objection* . . . An objection is an 'all-things-considered' judgement because the cons outweigh any pros. As Buchanan (2011) notes, 'all objections are concerns, but not all concerns are objections' (p. 71).

References

Atzmon, G., Schechter, C., Greiner, W., Davidson, D., Rennert, G., & Barzilai, N. (2004). Clinical phenotype of families with longevity. *Journal of the American Geriatrics Society (JAGS)*, 52(2), 274–277. https://doi.org/10.1111/j.1532-5415.2004.52068.x
Austad, S. (2006). Why women live longer than men: Sex differences in longevity. *Gender Medicine*, 3, 79–92.
Austad, S. N. (1997). *Why we age*. John Wiley.
Barbi, E., Lagona, F., Marsili, M., Vaupel, J. W., & Wachter, K. W. (2018). The plateau of human mortality: Demography of longevity pioneers. *Science (American Association for the Advancement of Science)*, 360(6396), 1459–1461. https://doi.org/10.1126/science.aat3119
Barzilai, N., Crandall, J. P., Kritchevsky, S. B., & Espeland, M. A. (2016). Metformin as a tool to target aging. *Cell Metabolism*, 23(6), 1060–1065. https://doi.org/10.1016/j.cmet.2016.05.011
Broskey, N. T., Marlatt, K. L., Most, J., Erickson, M. L., Irving, B. A., & Redman, L. M. (2019). The panacea of human aging: Calorie restriction versus exercise.

Exercise and Sport Sciences Reviews, *47*(3), 169–175. https://doi.org/10.1249/JES.0000000000000193

Buchanan, A. (2011). *Beyond humanity*. Oxford University Press.

Butler, R. N. (1969). Age-ism: Another form of bigotry. *The Gerontologist*, *9*(1), 243–246.

Butler, R. N., Miller, R. A., Perry, D., Carnes, B. A., Williams, T. F., Cassel, C., Brody, J., Bernard, M. A., Partridge, L., Kirkwood, T., Martin, G. M., & Olshansky, S. J. (2008). New model of health promotion and disease prevention for the 21st century. *British Medical Journal*, *337*(7662), e125–e150. https://doi.org/10.1136/bmj.a399

Carnes, B. A. (2007). Senescence viewed through the lens of comparative biology. *Annals of the New York Academy of Sciences*, *1114*(1), 14–22. https://doi.org/10.1196/annals.1396.045

Carnes, B. A., Olshansky, S. J., & Grahn, D. (2003). Biological evidence for limits to the duration of life. *Biogerontology (Dordrecht)*, *4*(1), 31–45. https://doi.org/10.1023/A:1022425317536

Ellis, S., Franks, D. W., Nattrass, S., Cant, M. A., Bradley, D. L., Giles, D., Balcomb, K. C., & Croft, D. P. (2018). Postreproductive lifespans are rare in mammals. *Ecology and Evolution*, *8*(5), 2482–2494. https://doi.org/10.1002/ece3.3856

Evert, J., Lawler, E., Bogan, H., & Perls, T. (2003). Morbidity profiles of centenarians: Survivors, delayers, and escapers. *The Journals of Gerontology. Series A, Biological Sciences and Medical Sciences*, *58*(3), M232–M237. https://doi.org/10.1093/gerona/58.3.M232

Fahy, G. M., Brooke, R. T., Watson, J. P., Good, Z., Vasanawala, S. S., Maecker, H., Leipold, M. D., Lin, D. T. S., Kobor, M. S., & Horvath, S. (2019). Reversal of epigenetic aging and immunosenescent trends in humans. *Aging Cell*, *18*(6), e13028. https://doi.org/10.1111/acel.13028

Farrelly, C. P. (2023a). Longevity science and women's health and wellbeing. *Journal of Population Ageing (Advance Online)*, 1–20. https://doi.org/10.1007/s12062-023-09411-y

Farrelly, C. P. (2023b). Geroscience and climate science: Oppositional or complementary? *Aging Cell (Advance Online)*, e13890. https://doi.org/10.1111/acel.13890

Franco, O. H., de Laet, C., Peeters, A., Jonker, J., Mackenbach, J., & Nusselder, W. (2005). Effects of physical activity on life expectancy with cardiovascular disease. *Archives of Internal Medicine (1960)*, *165*(20), 2355–2360. https://doi.org/10.1001/archinte.165.20.2355

Fries, J. F. (2005). The compression of morbidity. *The Milbank Quarterly*, *83*(4), 801–823. https://doi.org/10.1111/j.1468-0009.2005.00401.x

Gurven, M., & Kaplan, H. (2007). Longevity among hunter- gatherers: A cross-cultural examination. *Population and Development Review*, *33*(2), 321–365. https://doi.org/10.1111/j.1728-4457.2007.00171.x

Hamilton, J., & Mestler, G. (1969). Mortality and survival: Comparison of eunuchs with intact men and women in a mentally retarded population. *Journal of Gerontology*, *24*(4), 395–411.

Harrison, D. E., Strong, R., Sharp, Z. D., Nelson, J. F., Astle, C. M., Flurkey, K., Nadon, N. L., Wilkinson, J. E., Frenkel, K., Carter, C. S., Pahor, M., Javors, M. A., Fernandez, E., & Miller, R. A. (2009). Rapamycin fed late in life extends lifespan in genetically heterogeneous mice. *Nature*, *460*(7253), 392–395. https://doi.org/10.1038/nature08221

Hayflick, L. (2003). *Has anyone ever died of old age?* International Longevity Centre.

Holliday, R. (1999). Ageing in the 21st century. *The Lancet, 354,* SIV4.

Holloszy, J., & Fontana, L. (2007). Caloric restriction in humans. *Experimental Gerontology, 42*(8), 709–712.

Kaeberlein, M., Rabinovitch, P. S., & Martin, G. M. (2015). Healthy aging: The ultimate preventative medicine. *Science (American Association for the Advancement of Science), 350*(6265), 1191–1193. https://doi.org/10.1126/science.aad3267

Karlsson, E. K., Kwiatkowski, D. P., & Sabeti, P. C. (2014). Natural selection and infectious disease in human populations. *Nature Reviews. Genetics, 15*(6), 379–393. https://doi.org/10.1038/nrg3734

Kennedy, B. K., Berger, S. L., Brunet, A., Campisi, J., Cuervo, A. M., Epel, E. S., Franceschi, C., Lithgow, G. J., Morimoto, R. I., Pessin, J. E., Rando, T. A., Richardson, A., Schadt, E. E., Wyss-Coray, T., & Sierra, F. (2014). Geroscience: Linking aging to chronic disease. *Cell, 159*(4), 709–713. https://doi.org/10.1016/j.cell.2014.10.039

Kirkwood, T. B. (1977). Evolution of aging. *Nature, 270,* 301–304.

Kirkwood, T. B., & Austad, S. (2000). Why do we age? *Nature, 408*(9), 233–238.

Kirkwood, T. B., & Holliday, R. (1979). The evolution of ageing and longevity. *Proceedings of the Royal Society of London: Biology, 205,* 531–546.

Kirkwood, T. B., & Melov, S. (2011). On the programmed/non-programmed nature of ageing within the life history. *Current Biology, 21*(18), R701–R707. https://doi.org/10.1016/j.cub.2011.07.020

Koplow, D. (2003). *Smallpox: The fight to eradicate a global scourge.* University of California Press.

Kowald, A., & Kirkwood, T. (2016). Can aging be programmed? A critical literature review. *Aging Cell, 15,* 986–998.

Le Couteur, D., Anderson, R., & de Cabo, R. (2018). Sex and aging. *Journals of Gerontology: Biological Sciences, 73*(2), 139–140.

Medawar, P. (1952). *An unsolved problem of biology.* Lewis.

Miller, R. (2002). Extending life: Scientific prospects and political obstacles. *The Milbank Quarterly, 80*(1), 155–174.

Min, K.-J., Lee, C.-K., & Park, H.-N. (2012). The lifespan of Korean eunuchs. *Current Biology, 22*(18), R792–R793. https://doi.org/10.1016/j.cub.2012.06.036

Nesse, R. (2019). *Good reasons for bad feelings: Insights from the frontier of evolutionary psychiatry.* Penguin Random House.

Nesse, R., & Williams, G. (1996). *Why we get sick: The new science of Darwinian medicine.* Vintage Books.

NIH. (2022, April 04). *Progeria gene implicated in normal aging.* www.nih.gov/news-events/nih-research-matters/progeria-gene-implicated-normal-aging#

Novelle, M. G., Ali, A., Diéguez, C., Bernier, M., & de Cabo, R. (2016). Metformin: A hopeful promise in aging research. *Cold Spring Harbor Perspectives in Medicine, 6*(3), a025932–a025932. https://doi.org/10.1101/cshperspect.a025932

Olshansky, S. J. (2018). From lifespan to healthspan. *The Journal of the American Medical Association, 320*(13), 1323–1324.

Olshansky, S. J., Carnes, B., & Cassel, C. (1990). In search of Methuselah: Estimating the upper limits to human longevity. *Science (American Association for the Advancement of Science), 250*(4981), 634–640. https://doi.org/10.1126/science.2237414

Olshansky, S. J., Carnes, B., & Cassel, C. (1993). The aging of the human species. *Scientific American, 268,* 46–52.

Palmore, E. (1999). *Ageism: Negative and positive* (2nd ed.). Springer Publishing Company.

Perls, T. T., Bubrick, E., Wager, C. G., Vijg, J., & Kruglyak, L. (1998). Siblings of centenarians live longer. *The Lancet (British Edition)*, *351*(9115), 1560–1560. https://doi.org/10.1016/S0140-6736(05)61126-9

Racette, S. B., Weiss, E. P., Villareal, D. T., Arif, H., Steger-May, K., Schechtman, K. B., Fontana, L., Klein, S., & Holloszy, J. O. (2006). One year of caloric restriction in humans: Feasibility and effects on body composition and abdominal adipose tissue. *The Journals of Gerontology. Series A, Biological Sciences and Medical Sciences*, *61*(9), 943–950. https://doi.org/10.1093/gerona/61.9.943

Rose, M. (2005). *The long tomorrow: How advances in evolutionary biology can help us postpone aging*. Oxford University Press.

Scott-Phillips, T., Dickins, T., & West, S. (2011). Evolutionary theory and the ultimate – Proximate distinction in the human behavioral sciences. *Perspectives on Psychological Science*, *6*(1), 38–47.

Singer, M. (2016). The origins of aging: Evidence that aging is an adaptive phenotype. *Current Aging Science*, *9*(2), 95–115.

Tabatabaie, V., Atzmon, G., Rajpathak, S. N., Freeman, R., Barzilai, N., & Crandall, J. (2011). Exceptional longevity is associated with decreased reproduction. *Aging (Albany, NY.)*, *3*(12), 1202–1205. https://doi.org/10.18632/aging.100415

Taylor, L. H., Latham, S. M., & Woolhouse, M. E. (2001). Risk factors for human disease emergence. *Philosophical Transactions. Biological Sciences*, *356*(1411), 983–989. https://doi.org/10.1098/rstb.2001.0888

Unicef. (2022, April 21). *Unicef's game plan to end open defecation*. www.unicef.org/documents/unicefs-game-plan-end-open-defecation

United Nations, Department of Economic and Social Affairs & Population Division. (2012). *World Mortality Report 2011* (United Nations publication). https://www.un.org/en/development/desa/population/publications/pdf/mortality/worldMortalityReport2011.pdf

Vogeli, C., Shields, A. E., Lee, T. A., Gibson, T. B., Marder, W. D., Weiss, K. B., & Blumenthal, D. (2007). Multiple chronic conditions: Prevalence, health consequences, and implications for quality, care management, and costs. *Journal of General Internal Medicine: JGIM*, *22*(S3), 391–395. https://doi.org/10.1007/s11606-007-0322-1

Weissmann, A. (1891). *Essays on heredity*. Clarendon Press.

Weon, B. M., & Je, J. H. (2009). Theoretical estimation of maximum human lifespan. *Biogerontology (Dordrecht)*, *10*(1), 65–71. https://doi.org/10.1007/s10522-008-9156-4

WHO Programme on Ageing and Health, Division of Health Promotion, Education and Communication. (1997). The Brasilia declaration on ageing. *Health Promotion International*, *12*(2), 175–178.

3 Anti-Aging or Enhancing-Aging Technologies?

Social and Religious Implications of Radical Life Extension

Tracy J. Trothen

Introduction

Life-extension technologies are already very profitable and sought after. Most of us want to avoid death for as long as possible provided that we can maintain our minds, bodies, and loved ones. This chapter considers significant ethical issues regarding possible social implications of emerging life enhancement and radical life-extending technologies.

The United Nations Population Fund (UNFPA) reported that the global population of individuals over the age of 60 totalled 841 million in 2013. By 2050, this number is projected to increase to two billion. One in five Canadians probably will be 65 or older in 2024. As of July 1, 2018, according to Statistics Canada (2019), almost one in two older adults (46.3%) were born during the baby boom period. This proportion has increased rapidly, up from 41.3% one year earlier (Statistics Canada, 2019). The World Health Organization (2019) notes that the "global average life expectancy increased by 5 years [to 71.4 years] between 2000 and 2015, the fastest increase since the 1960s". We are living longer and the percentage of people 65 and older is increasing quickly.

At the same time, the pace of technological developments is also accelerating, possibly soon allowing us to "outrun our own deaths", as well-known futurist, inventor, and computer scientist Ray Kurzweil contends (Holman, 2013). Scientist Aubrey de Grey (2009) and other superlongevity proponents call this acceleration "longevity escape velocity" (LEV). When we reach LEV, we will be able to extend our lives long enough for the next needed technological breakthrough. That breakthrough will then allow us to extend our lives again until the next breakthrough, thus allowing us to escape or outrun death. Interestingly, Kurzweil became the director of engineering for Google in 2012. Shortly after Kurzweil's appointment, Google launched a project called Calico with the purpose of studying health and aging and "to solve death" (McCracken & Grossman, 2013). Kurzweil since became a principal researcher and A.I. visionary at Google.

This chapter begins with a brief exploration of the moral relevance of values and social processes that influence desire and choice, then provides a brief overview of some existing, emerging and aspiring technologies to extend life.

DOI: 10.4324/9781032617282-4

Next three main ethical issues are presented. The first ethical issue concerns the anthropological question of what it means to be human. Much ethical analysis has relied on a therapy/enhancement distinction with therapies considered morally "good" and enhancements not so good since they take us beyond an accepted state of "normal". Do interventions that stop or even reverse bodily aging bring us back to normal, or do they enhance us beyond what or who we should be? The second ethical issue that will be discussed is morphological freedom of choice. In Canada, much attention is being given to the freedom to choose assisted death (Browne & Russell, 2016). What about the freedom to choose assisted life through radical life-extending technologies? The moral relevance of interdependence, social processes, and ageism are considered. The third ethical issue is social justice, including systemic marginalization and resource allocation. Finally, the chapter concludes by examining the power of words to shape ethical discourse. "Anti-aging technologies" suggests that interventions to extend life or mitigate manifestations of aging are against not only aging but may be the aged, whereas "human enhancement technologies" suggests ways to make us better.

Values and Social Processes

This chapter considers radical life extension from the perspective of an ethicist who specializes in theology and ethics. The questions explored in this chapter are situated in the reality that everyone brings values and commitments to ethical analyses. These values and commitments are continually shaped by multivariant sources including personal experiences, families of origin, news and social media, research, politics, regulatory bodies, and religions. These values and commitments are aspects of our individual viewpoints from which we approach ethical issues.

Taking an intersectional approach, committed to the inclusion and prioritizing of socially and politically marginalized people, some of the implications of "anti-aging" technologies for diverse people over the age of 65 are considered here. An intersectional theological lens is used in this chapter to begin to identify justice concerns. Intersectional theology emphasizes the impact of interlocking systemic privilege and power on experience and ways of seeing the world. Theologians Grace Ji-Sun Kim and Susan M. Shaw (2018) explain that:

> . . . the further from the norm, the greater the marginalization. This marginalization, however, is not simply additive, but rather social categories of gender, race, class, and other forms of difference interact with and shape one another within interconnected systems of oppression. These systems of oppression – sexism, racism, colonialism, classism, ableism, nativism, and ageism – work within social institutions such as education, work, religion, and the family . . . to structure our experiences and relationships in such a way that we participate in reproducing dominance and subordination without even realizing it.
>
> (p. 1)

Perhaps the most obvious systemic barrier relevant to this book is ageism. The undervaluing and stigmatizing of older adults is prevalent in mainstream North America. Unless you fit into a "successful aging" paradigm by continuing to be measurably productive, well off financially and to all appearances independent, you risk becoming regarded as insignificant at best or a burden and a drain on society at worst (Holstein et al., 2011). Many people experience being discounted, not heard, talked down to, or otherwise devalued as they develop visible signs of aging like grey hair, wrinkles, or more limited mobility. A stunning example of ageism which demonstrates the appeal of a technological cure was the Kia commercial unveiled during the 2018 Super Bowl. As Aerosmith's 1973 hit "Dream On" plays in the background, lead singer 69-year-old Steven Tyler races a new Kia Stinger and becomes young again. Kia's tagline in the commercial was "Feel something again". The implication is that as we age we lose vibrancy and become irrelevant and boring, unable to be stimulated and engaged. Technology promises to make us young again; old, boring, and dull are avoided. We are told what we really want: youthful and exciting tech. And we are told what we really don't want: aging, dependence, and vulnerability.

An evolutionary perspective shows that we tend to desire things that fail to satisfy us for long. Acquisitions lead to the desire for more. Unearthing what we really want, if we really want something that provides long-term satisfaction, remains elusive for many people (Hopkins, 2015). Part of the reason for this persistent elusiveness are the many social processes that are in place to shape what we think we want. Relational theorists, such as ethicist Susan Sherwin, detail the complexities of these social processes (Sherwin, 2012). There are many ways in which we are told what we desire. Social media, TV, and advertisements tell us how we should look and what we should buy if we want to be successful and happy. Science sometimes tells us what is normal and what is aberrant. Political leaders often tell us what is best for our country and the world. And so on. Much of the input we receive is informative and constructive. Much of it serves particular interests such as profit for big business, votes for elected officials, or self-protection. Figuring out what is most important to us, and what we really want, is no easy task.

Technology and Values

Complicating things even more, technology itself propagates values. European philosophers such as Marcuse (1964), Habermas (1971), and Foucault (1988) have uncovered social processes that have led to the false belief that technology is value-neutral. Technology itself promotes the values of utility and efficiency. Smartwatches help us to be more efficient at responding to phone calls, texts, and emails. Dishwashers mean that we spend less time washing and drying dishes. Microwaves reduce cooking time. Power tools hasten building projects and repairs. Robots make it easier and reduce the number of human caregivers needed, to comfort distressed or lonely people – including the elderly (Purtill, 2019). ChatGPT not only gives us information and does student assignments (or at least tries) but this and other generative algorithms also provide support, jokes, and/or responses to just about any question. We need to ask if there is a point at which we lose something through the increased use of technology. Some suggest that increased technology can reduce opportunities for happiness by taking away day-to-day challenges; the successful completion of small, doable challenges generates happiness and the possibility of experiencing wonder (Feezell, 2013; Dreyfus & Kelly, 2011). Given our human need for challenges, might our capacity for wonder, awe, hope, and relationship become more limited if we reduce more aspects of our lives to technologically executed tasks (Dreyfus & Kelly, 2011)? On the other hand, maybe other meaningful challenges and relationships will be created through technology. Nonetheless, we need to be attentive to the effect that increasing technology has on our everyday lives including our happiness and our values.

Values "pertain to beliefs and attitudes that provide direction to everyday living" (Corey et al., 2015, p. 14) and are those things that are most important to us. Values inform our ideals for living. Examples of values are achievement, integrity, relationships, justice, loyalty, power, pleasure, and wisdom. Values do not automatically inform our desires. We need to be intentional in examining what is most important to each of us. Our values should be deliberately engaged when we think about ethics issues including aging and superlongevity. Consider taking 10–15 minutes to identify your top five values. Try not to overthink this; there is no "right" answer. If you're having trouble identifying your values, ask yourself what you want to be remembered for. What do you want your obituary to say?

Once we identify our values, self-reflexivity – "the process of reflecting on one's own story from multiple diverging standpoints in ways that try to take into account one's own experience of privilege and disadvantage within intersecting social systems like sexism, racism, heterosexism, and religious forms of oppression" (Doehring, 2015, p. 191) – is the next step. To understand what we really want and how best to get what we really want, we also need to understand what we have and what we experience systemically. Social systems affect our identities, our experiences, and our values and desires. Understanding that not everyone is treated equitably in society and that our treatment is influenced by racialization, gender and sexual identity bias, socio-economic status, ableism, and other factors can illuminate the moral relevance of systemic power imbalances. Not everyone is valued equally. We are taught to aspire to become part of the most valued social groups, when what we really need is to critique these power imbalances and systems of oppression in which some are seen as less valuable than others. Self-reflexivity helps us to recognize and critique normative values. In this way, we can begin to understand more deeply what it is that we might choose to value if we were not formed by often complex and subtle social processes.

Anti-Aging Biohacks and Technologies

As discussed in earlier chapters, anti-aging biohacks and technologies range from therapies such as severe calorie restriction, plastic surgery, and exercise programs, to emerging technologies such as new stem cell therapies, gene therapies and gene editing, brain–computer interfaces (BCIs), robotics, and other cybernetics (e.g., cochlear implants, pacemakers, artificial retinas, prosthetic limbs, and exoskeletons). Nanotechnology, replacement organs, cell regeneration, cryogenics, and whole brain emulation are considered more fantastical, yet advances are being made on all these fronts. On the simpler end, face creams and other treatment regimens for skin wrinkles can be considered as an anti-aging intervention (Holstein et al., 2011). De Grey (2009) adds immunotherapies and glycation link-breakers (which may hold the key to many age-related diseases) to this list.

Gene therapies have been launched and are expanding. Although at the time it was still only a phase 2 drug therapy, in August 2017, Kymriah was fast tracked, becoming the first gene therapy (using viral transfection, not CRISPR) to receive FDA approval in the United States. Almost exactly one year later, Kymriah was approved by Health Canada. Kymriah is a drug composed of a patient's own genetically modified immune cells (T-cells) for the treatment of B-cell acute lymphoblastic leukaemia (ALL). ALL is a deadly form of childhood blood cancer. One study reports that 83% of ALL patients achieve full remission within three months of receiving the gene therapy (Seger, 2017). Kymriah is now also being used to treat a form of adult non-Hodgkin's lymphoma, but the treatment can be very expensive. Similarly, another very expensive gene therapy, Luxterna, was given FDA approval in late 2017[1] for the treatment of congenital blindness resulting from a genetic mutation in the *RPE65* gene, which causes degenerative retinal disease. More gene therapies have since become available in different countries, including a treatment for certain types of bladder cancer, a treatment for certain kinds of haemophilia B and Vyjuvek (a vector-based gene therapy) for the treatment of wounds in people with a type of dystrophic epidermolysis (DEB) which was approved by the US FDA in 2023.

With the development of Clustered Regularly Interspaced Short Palindromic Repeats (CRISPR) technology in 2012, it became easier to edit genomes. CRISPR/Cas9 is now being used in gene therapies to reverse Huntington's symptoms in mice. Companies such as Editas are promising competition for Sparks (the owner of Luxterna) with the development of a CRISPR/Cas9 treatment for the same congenital blindness condition. Treatments for diseases (e.g., B-thalassemia and sickle cell disease) are also under development using CRISPR technology (Sheridan, 2020).

Strides are also being made towards gene therapies that treat aging-related health issues. These include repairing brain tissue damaged by stroke and improving memory and motor skills beyond the pre-stroke level (Collins, 2019); treating cardiovascular disease in mice (Smith, 2019); and decelerating the aging process in mice with Hutchinson–Gilford progeria syndrome, a rare genetic disorder that accelerates the aging process (Beyret et al., 2019) and which also occurs in humans. Even though aging itself cannot be addressed through one specific gene (Holstein et al., 2011), there are promising indicators that gene therapies could extend lives, and for some people already are.

What Does It Mean to Be Human?

Is aging a disease that we should try to prevent? Or should we aim only for compressed morbidity? There is the danger that we will blindly work towards "curing" aging. By this, I mean that simply because we can extend, or even radically extend, human life, we will. It may be that we arrive at this same conclusion – that life should be extended as much as possible – after we intentionally explore relevant ethical issues. Even if we arrive at this same conclusion, however, we may decide to approach the issue of aging differently than we are now.

The questions of what it means to be human and what is valuable about being human are important to this conversation about radical life extension. Ought we try to alter "human nature"? Is there an essential human nature? While many agree that there is no one essential and defining dimension of being human, there are themes or qualities that most regard as desirable human aspects. Two of these aspects are embodiment, and the capacity to be virtuous. Even these aspects are not beyond debate; some say that there are alternative ways to be embodied that could allow us to live forever. One argument is that we do not have to be fleshy bodies but could be integrated into a computer substrate as a body. Regarding virtue, we are developing science that may allow (some of?) us to become more virtuous by being less aggressive, more altruistic and empathetic. But these moral enhancement technologies are not beyond debate. Who decides what it means to be virtuous? Does everyone need more of the same qualities to be better morally? Marginalized groups, for example, may not need more empathy or to be more self-sacrificing; they may instead need more assertiveness and even aggression (Trothen, 2017, Mercer & Trothen, 2021).

With the acceleration in technological means to make us better, we need to ask more directly what it is that we value about being human and if we even want to remain human. These questions may seem shocking but the reality is that what it means to be human has shifted over the centuries and will continue to shift – likely at an increasing pace.

What is considered "normal" shifts according to time and context. What might seem outlandish or even offensive to some of us now, may come to be normal in the future. Consider that until the 1950s, it was seen as the height (or depth) of hubris to tamper with the human heart. When the first successful blue baby surgery occurred at Johns Hopkins Hospital in 1944 that attitude began to change.[2] Not too many years later, heart surgeries became "normal" procedures. Gene therapies are becoming more normal. Radical life extension may also become normal and be seen as part of being human or post-human.

Arguments based on an essentialist understanding of being human and not an evolutionary concept of being are limited to a here and now context and to whomever it is that is defining the human experience.

The dynamism of normal complicates an approach to medical interventions that tries to distinguish therapy from enhancement. In this approach, the dividing line is whatever is regarded as normal, with therapies seen as those interventions that may bring us to normal and interventions that enhance us, or bring us beyond what is considered normal, as abnormal. However, just because this is a complicated approach, this approach is still useful as a first guide to deciding which medical interventions ought to be prioritized. As we will discuss later in this chapter, we live in a world of limited resources. For that reason alone, we need to have some way to prioritize the most needed medical interventions. Those interventions that have clear therapeutic value supersede the value of interventions that make life better than what might be considered normal. For example, coronary artery bypass grafting is needed to prevent some people with heart disease from dying. Laser eye surgery to improve someone's sight past 20/20 is an enhancing intervention, designed to improve eyesight beyond what is commonly accepted as normal. While better than 20/20 vision may be nice to have, it is not necessary to life.

If part of being human is an ability to value life, we need to ask if life will be valued more or less in a "post-aging world". Some will anticipate no change in how we value life. Others might say that more time will give us more opportunity to value life and to do good works, while others believe that it is the knowledge of our mortality that motivates us to live well and attempt to make the world a better place. According to Vail and colleagues (2012),

> [t]he awareness of mortality can motivate people to enhance their physical health and prioritize growth-oriented goals; live up to positive standards and beliefs; build supportive relationships and encourage the development of peaceful, charitable communities; and foster open-minded and growth-oriented behaviors.
>
> (p. 303)

Attitudes towards death and dying are crucial to conversations about being human and aging. The values that we hold and contextual factors, such as culture, influence how we view aging, dying, and death. Cultures that view death as a normal and defining moment of life may also see aging less as a scary thing to be avoided at all costs and more as a respected life stage. For example, Indigenous cultures view dying as a rite of passage as elders enter the spirit world to be alongside the creator (Hampton et al., 2010). In contrast, many non-Indigenous North Americans are more inclined to focus on maintaining the appearance of youthfulness and denying mortality (Holstein et al., 2011).

Connected to a shift away from seeing dying as a natural and inevitable process to medicalizing the aging process, many of us have avoided and denied death (Waldrop, 2011). In spite of the hospice movement, led by Dame Cicely Saunders in the 1960s, in North America, talk of death is mostly avoided and death remains largely hidden (e.g., Bregman, 1999). But talking about death can help us to see death as part of life, and perhaps slowly change our views about aging and death (Hanning, 2017). Death Cafés are one way to start the conversation and change perspectives on mortality. These groups are run on a voluntary basis and encourage people to come to terms with death, make the most of their lives, and avoid existential angst. Such conversations may change the way we think about death and aging.

If we were not as terrified of death or in denial about death and dying, would we be as enthusiastic about eradicating aging and mortality? Transhumanists, especially, see aging and death as our biggest enemies that need defeating (Herzfeld, 2017; Mercer & Trothen, 2021). Through technology, we may be able to radically extend life to the point that we will only die from accidents, murder, climate change, or cosmic events such as meteorites or planet death. Will we get what we want by making it possible to live to 500 or longer? It is possible that when we think more deliberately about death, some of us will become more passionate about radical life extension. Some may say that radical life extension would be wonderful so long as our quality of life is good and the ones we love are still alive, too. Others "may feel that they have reached a stage of completion in their lives at a certain age" (Ekerdt et al., 2017, p. 46). For now, as we age, we come closer to death. The uncertainty of life beyond death, and the spiritual and religious views an individual may possess, influences desires to live longer (Hallberg, 2004).

Many religions do not believe that death is the end. Karmic religions hold that souls are reincarnated. Monotheistic traditions believe in the possibility of heaven. A belief that there is life after death ought not to make people want to die – since life is seen as a gift from God – but it does provide reassurance that there is more, even if the more is unknown. An article by the Pew Research Center (2013) on *Religious Leaders' Views on Radical Life Extension* found that most religious leaders surveyed supported both life enhancement and extension – provided that it did not result in immortality and the avoidance of death. The alleviation of suffering is clearly in line with Judeo-Christian philosophies (Herzfeld, 2017, p. 291) but the dread of physical death is not. From a monotheistic perspective, attempts to create our own immortality, to re-create ourselves in our own image, are borne of a failure to recognize the limitedness of human capability. Humans are not perfect. For perfection, monotheistic religions look to a transcendent God. As theologian Phil Hefner (2009) cautions,

Essential human nature is violated when we obliterate or no longer acknowledge the sense that we are accountable to something larger than ourselves and larger than our own times. . . . Our humanity is compromised when we forget that our personhood is defined in the engagement with this something larger.

(p. 165)

The question of where we might find immortality and salvation loom large in the backdrop of aging and technological salvation. The Islamic and Judeo-Christian traditions all involve some narrative that includes resurrection and endless life with God. Are immortality and salvation to be found in technology? In religion? Or perhaps in both? Technology alone cannot give us life everlasting. We live in an impermanent planet and universe. As Protestant theologian Ron Cole-Turner (2009) puts it, "Technology offers to give us what we want, or at least what most of us think we want – longer life, youthful bodies, greater health, and mental ability. Christianity invites us to give up what we want, indeed to give up life itself, as the one condition for real life" (p. 58).

But this does not mean that religion is inconsistent with life-extension, and even radical life-extension, technologies. Part of religious mandates is to do good. Doing good is usually understood to include healing and helping people to live healthy and happy lives. The commandments to "Love the Lord your God with all your heart and with all your soul and with all your mind" and "Love your neighbour as yourself" are central to Jewish and Christian theologies. As such, the duty to do good is more than aspirational. Insofar as science and technology are used to do people good, religion is supportive. But the question of what it means to do good is complex.

As technological developments accelerate, we have more decisions to make concerning how to re-create ourselves. While improving health and relieving suffering are consistent with Judeo-Christian theological beliefs, how might a belief in the intrinsic goodness of diverse embodied people affect how we see enhancing technologies? In the award-winning documentary film, Fixed (2013) explores how ableist attitudes affect what aspects of being human are assumed to need to be fixed or changed since these aspects are not valued in normative circles. The belief that we are valued primarily for being instead of for our utility also may impact the enhancing technologies we choose to pursue. Moreover, if death is not seen as the worst thing and may even be seen as accompanying hope for life everlasting or life reincarnated, then the meaning of living well may not require living forever. On the other hand, if more good can be done or more pleasure experienced, then radical life extension could potentially be embraced as a good thing.

Weighing the potential harms and benefits of radical life extension, in terms of what it means to be human, is complicated. Much of what it means to be human has to do with the values we hold. What do we most value about being human? What do we want to change? For aging adults, there could be pressure to avoid aging because of the implications that aging has for our perceived worth. And there is pressure to want to look young, act young, and, generally, not be old. In some cultures, aging is seen as giving us the opportunity to be purveyors of wisdom. Worldviews, including religion, and prejudices, such as ageism, sexism, and racialization, affect perceptions of what it means to be human and to be desirable humans.

Medical interventions that stop or change aging may become seen as necessary therapies, not enhancements. If aging is seen as an unnecessary disease instead of a normal, necessary, and valued aspect of being human, then we will likely choose radical life-extending technologies as these become available. It may be that even if we get past ageism, we still want to live for much longer because we value this life. But who gets to choose and how do we choose?

Choice, Extreme Individualism, and Social Processes

The individual right to make choices is highly valued in North American society, and morphological freedom is highly valued by anti-aging proponents (Labrecque, 2015). It may seem straightforward: I can choose life-extending technologies as they emerge, or not. End of story. But it is not that simple.

First, not everyone is judged as able to make choices on their own. If the questions of anti-aging technologies and radical life extension are all about individual choice, this potentially leaves out those with cognitive impairment including aging adults with dementia or Alzheimer's disease. Again, we have to ask who should have access to life-extending technologies? As long as individual rights and rational choice are highly valued in North America, the focus remains on individual financial resources and the legal capacity to think for oneself.

Second, our preoccupation with individual rights can shift attention away from responsibility and make it difficult to see that a person's choice to live longer, or not, does not only affect that person. While individual rights are important, so too is responsibility for communal and global well-being. We will look further at this social justice aspect of responsibility and rights in the next section.

Third, connected to the rights or responsibility emphasis is the moral relevance of context. Personal decisions about life-extending technologies do not operate in a vacuum. Individual choices are not made independent of contextual factors, including social processes (Sherwin, 2012). Worldwide, many societies value collectivity and relationships, respect for elders, religion, and harmony. In contrast, large proportions of Western societies prize individualism, self-sufficiency, autonomy, and production (Mazanah & Merriam, 2000). There is a general attitude in North America that frames "successful aging" in terms of ongoing productivity and independent functioning (Holstein et al., 2011). It is easy to forget that we are all interdependent and rely on others. When asked to think about how they get a new laptop or iPhone, students will often answer that it is just a "click" away. But numerous people are involved in getting that new tech to us: delivery people, people involved in packaging, computer scientists, and business administrators. Just about everything we do involves someone else.

A cultural denigration of dependence only serves to mask and deny this interdependent reality. As aging adults often become less mobile, their need for others becomes more visible. Added to this increase in visible need, they may become more conscious about mortality. Awareness that we will die means admitting our finiteness. Dependence and finiteness are features of being human that are not valued in "mainstream" North America. But just because dependence and mortality are unpopular does not mean that they are not real or that they are without value.

As ethicists Martha Holstein and her colleagues (2011) note in their examination of ethics and aging, "[d]ependence has been associated with weakness, incapacity, neediness, and a lack of dignity" (p. 12). If we take a more intentional approach to dependence, we can see that all life is dependent on other life. But if we are invested in denying that interdependence, then it can come as an unpleasant shock when we encounter life situations in which we are confronted by our need for others. If we cannot even acknowledge our everyday interdependence, then it becomes very difficult to accept the times when we must ask for or receive help. Agich (2003) in his ethical analysis of autonomy and long-term care home residents concludes that human dependency is valuable and "non-accidental" (p. 605), going on to explain that dependency brings us into relationship with each other. Awareness that we are not sufficient alone can help us to see the intrinsic value and dignity of the other (Holstein et al., 2011).

Attitudes towards aging influence our identities, desires, and choices. If dependence is seen as weakness and is associated with being a burden, then we are more apt to choose options that may lessen dependency. Similarly, a fear of death and dying will likely steer us in the direction of radical life extension when and if these measures become available, even if there are potential harms. As it stands, there are indeed serious risks associated with many emerging anti-aging technologies. For example, the long-term implications of germ-line editing are unknown. And of course, there are consent issues involved in any decision to change germ-line cells since future generations will also be affected. Some gene therapies, including some using CRISPR/Cas9, appear promising and yet, these therapies are in their infancy, and we do not know what the long-term risks may be. Given that our values are influenced by social processes and attitudes, it remains very difficult to know what we want. With accelerating advancements in technology, it is becoming even more pressing to choose first to take a deliberate look at the values we hold and the social processes that inform these values. Then we can decide which, if any, anti-aging technologies we want.

While many may choose radical life-extending technologies, some would not. Some studies have shown that individuals only want to live longer if they are in good health (e.g., Donner et al., 2015). When given the choice, as Donner and colleagues discovered, some individuals would rather live an average lifespan as compared to an unlimited lifespan if aging means disease and lower quality of life.

Living healthier is not only related to physical well-being and the avoidance of disease but also encompasses cognitive, affective, and spiritual well-being (Burke et al., 2018). While many anti-aging technologies do not address all of these aspects (Ory et al., 2018), emerging radical life-extension and enhancement technologies do. It may be that eventually we will be able to radically extend life spans *and* make ourselves better physically, cognitively, affectively, spiritually, and even morally (Mercer & Trothen, 2021).

A religion can provide a lens through which particular values are encouraged and modelled. As with all religions, there are many interpretations of theologies but most would agree that love of neighbour and the recognition of the interdependence of all life are moral obligations. Responsibility, especially to those on the margins, is emphasized more than individual rights. Especially since some people's rights become more powerful than the rights of others due to layers of systemic oppression (e.g., because of ageism, racialization, ableism, sexual or gender identity, socio-economic status, and religion). Re-focusing on responsibility rather than individual rights can make room for equity.

If technology can enhance the possibility of living out these values, then in theory, it would be in keeping with many faith claims. On a cautionary note, as history attests, we have the capacity to make bad choices and do much harm, intended or not. Given human fallibility, a precautionary approach to radical life-extension technologies is important. On the other hand, many religious perspectives also strongly urge beneficence and recognize that the doing of good often entails some measure of risk.

Social Justice

The weight we give to potential social justice implications of life extension, both harms and benefits, needs to be weighed against morphological freedom of choice and what we value about being human. Possible social justice consequences of radical life extension include the following: a widening gap between the haves and have-nots; changes in human suffering; increased ageism; overpopulation or increased population; and ecological impacts.

In all likelihood, life-extending technologies will be prohibitively expensive for most people, at least when they are first introduced (Bagala, 2017). Kymriah and Luxterna, as discussed earlier, are good examples of the high costs of gene therapies. Since most radical life-extending interventions are not likely to be considered standard treatments in Canada, at least initially, it may be up to the individual to raise the funds. This means that the richer segment of society will have most access to life-extending and radical life-extending interventions which will likely result in them living longer and having the opportunity to accrue even more wealth. Proponents argue that although these technologies will be/are initially too expensive for most, they will quickly become affordable. However, even if this is true – which is very debatable – how much time will it take for the very wealthy to gain even more intractable social, political, and economic power by living longer? Moreover, the high costs allow private pharma corporations to capitalize on these technologies and gain even more wealth and power (Bagala, 2017). This corporate increase of wealth and power will have political implications; the countries with the greatest pharma gains will benefit in terms of political power. Almost certainly, the availability of radical life-extending technologies will significantly widen the global wealth gaps and the global power gaps.

On the other hand, aging is very "expensive to society and causes vast human suffering" (Holstein et al., 2011). Aging increases the risk of disease, chronic pain, and disability. Perhaps resources should be prioritized for the provision of emerging life-extension technologies as soon as they are approved for use. It is possible, theoretically, to decrease the long-term financial costs to our healthcare system by developing treatments that prevent or greatly lessen disease, physical disability, and pain. While these technologies may cost more initially, in the long run, they could save a lot of money. Also, just as many people practice preventative measures such as physical exercise and healthy eating, so that we may lessen our chances of disability and disease, should we not also have the option to do so through preventative anti-aging or superlongevity technologies?

However, while physical pain and decline *can* cause suffering, they do not always. Suffering is complicated. To lessen suffering, we need to determine the most significant causes of suffering associated with old age. Often the physical aspect of self is not the main cause of suffering. Suffering can be caused by emotional, cognitive, and spiritual distress. For instance, research has shown that some of the main reasons why people choose medically assisted death are the following: the loss of dignity, dependence and loss of control, being a burden, isolation and loneliness, uncertainty regarding one's future needs, overwhelming physical pain, hopelessness, and loss of meaning (Hendry et al., 2013). Those with fewer resources may have fewer choices for care and may be more likely to feel like a burden. Radical life-extending technologies may decrease suffering caused by physical issues such as pain, dependence, loss of dignity, and control. On the other hand, a change in societal attitude towards dependence may allow older adults to keep a sense of dignity when visibly dependent on others.

Radical life-extending technologies would not necessarily mitigate the suffering caused by loneliness, hopelessness, or loss of meaning. While greater longevity may well lessen physical suffering, it will not necessarily mitigate emotional, cognitive, and spiritual suffering. Systemic social inequities are at the root of significant suffering. Being ignored or attacked because you appear in a particular way that does not fit the "norm" causes suffering. Consider, for example, a disabled older woman who has scant financial resources because she had a lower paying job. It may be that her financial limitations prevent her from paying for extra care. Her care falls then to her adult children who already have pressure on them to care for their own children and hold down jobs. The older woman fears being a burden on the children she loves and cannot afford the latest non-standard therapies, so she petitions for medical assistance in dying (MAiD). Unless we address socioeconomic, geographic, racialization, ableism, ageism, and other inequities, it is very possible that radical life extension will amplify suffering rooted in or increased by these systemic barriers.

As longevity technology becomes available, people will likely be able to choose to radically extend their lives (if they have the finances) or not. But will there be a marginalizing of the unenhanced? Ageism may worsen if people can choose to avoid aging. Indeed, it may become regarded as a disease or disability and not as a normal part of living. In cultures in which the elderly are seen as very valuable and even revered, such as Indigenous, Indian, Greek, or Asian cultures (Löckenhoff et al., 2009), a decrease in visibly older adults may be disruptive. Alternately, appearance may take on lesser meaning if most people appear to be of a similar youthful age. Some scholars are convinced that radical life extension, and anti-aging medicine more generally, will heighten ageism (Holstein et al., 2011) towards those who choose to be unenhanced; older and even radically old people will not be discriminated against if they do not appear to be old. But we may discriminate increasingly against those who choose not, or cannot afford to choose, to use radical life-extending technologies and who opt to appear as aging and mortal adults. If invisible aging becomes the cultural norm, then our values will tend to align with the norm; cultural beliefs are important as they "shape social norms and values surrounding the aging process and the role of older people" (Chonody & Teater, 2018, n.p.).

Additional justice issues associated with possible radical life extension are overpopulation or increased population, and ecological impacts. Over-population is harming people and the earth especially in high-density urban locations. This problem likely will continue to worsen but optimistic proponents claim that we will develop technology that allows people to exist well in little physical space. For example, we are creating techniques to grow food faster and in very small spaces using hydroponics. In the meantime, however, we are polluting the earth at an alarming pace and creating social problems such as housing markets which are accessible only to the wealthy. Perhaps the colonization of space will present a possible solution, but should this represent the only possible solution?

Already we live longer in part due to therapeutic interventions (e.g., vaccines, exercise, healthy eating, joint replacements, and surgical interventions) that compress morbidity. While our goal is usually to compress morbidity, a result can be extended life. As *Harvard Gazette* contributor Alvin Powel puts it, "We can extend the lifespan of individuals not because we intentionally make them live longer, but because we are trying to help them avoid disease and stay healthy" (Powel, 2019). Earth's rapidly increasing population stretches resources such as physical space, healthcare, and education funding. More people means more waste and pollution. Climate change and eco-justice are moral imperatives if we value present and future life.

On the other hand, it may be the case that increasing population is a desirable outcome, indicating that we are collectively creating better living conditions and improved medical care. A few would argue that we do not want to make people's lives better and healthier. And we have demonstrated that people can learn to live in less space and more simply. But the tipping point may be climate change. Can we learn to live in ever-increasing numbers with a dramatically lower carbon footprint?

Many religions are very attentive to justice issues and the value and needs of the marginalized are prioritized. Many aging adults in North America are disadvantaged, and advocating for better elder care fits with many religious theologies. As a result, Christians, for example, may be suspicious of technologies that may result in the further margination of the visibly aging, even for the short term. On the other hand, healing is a strong theme in the scriptures associated with many religions. There are many biblical stories that promote healing, both on physical and spiritual levels.

Theologically, as created co-creators, humans remain inclined to both sin and to do good. The avoidance of sin is multi-pronged. Some theologians who examine human enhancement and technology emphasize the sin of pride or hubris. The admonition is not to play God. Others, such as Ted Peters and Ron Cole-Turner, are cautionary but exhort humanity to live more fully into our humanity by taking strategic risks to create for good and just purposes. Not all people are at as much risk of falling into the trap of hubris; others, who tend to be on the social margins, sin more through a lack of sufficient pride and self-love.

Moving Forward: What's in a Name and Where Do We Go From Here?

How we define an issue shapes the moral discourse that follows. Throughout this chapter, the following terms have been used: "anti-aging technologies", "radical life extension", "human enhancement", "transhumanism", "pro-longevity", and "superlongevity". While in some sense, these terms mean the same thing or at least significantly overlap in meaning, in other ways, they are very different.

As it reads on the American Academy of Religion website, regarding the Human Enhancement and Transhumanism Unit, "Transhumanism" or "human enhancement" refers to an intellectual and cultural movement that advocates the use of a variety of emerging technologies. The convergence of these technologies may make it possible to take control of human evolution, providing "'desirable' physical,[3] and the amelioration of aspects of the human condition regarded as undesirable. These enhancements include the radical extension of healthy human life". Similar to transhumanism and human enhancement, the terms "pro-longevity" and "superlongevity" connote positive and desirable goals and outcomes. "Radical life-extension" may stir both positive and negative responses, depending on how one feels about the term "radical". "Anti-aging technologies" or "anti-aging medicine" have more negative connotations, possibly indicating prejudice against aging adults.

Compounding the layers packed into these word choices are additional words that are used to explain technologies that may or do extend life. For example, "progress" suggests that technology is getting better and better. So too, the term "development". Scholars have critiqued these terms as they relate to technology and being human (Burdett, 2015). Science and religion scholar Michael Burdett suggests that "change" may be a better term since it does not assume the doctrinal faith claim that emerging technologies are *de facto* good. Another example are the words we use to define aging. Is aging a disease that ought to be cured? Is aging a normal and acceptable part of the human condition?

From an ethics perspective, it is important to be aware of the values and value judgements that may underlie these terms. The words we use to describe technology, like technology itself, can limit the questions we ask or can coerce us towards an implicit acceptance of certain values. Awareness of systemic privilege and disadvantage attached to age, culture, religion, racialization, socio-economic status, among others, and the moral relevance of these intersectional factors, must factor into any robust ethical discussion of radical life extension.

In the end, both proactive and precautionary approaches are needed in regard to the issue of radical life extension. Embedded beliefs, values, and desires must be identified and deliberately explored. We need to hear from diverse people if we are to understand the ways in which intersectional factors affect perspectives on and potential consequences of the use of technology to address aging. Worldviews and religions influence values and how ethical issues are perceived (Maher & Mercer, 2009; Mercer & Trothen, 2021). Faith-based perspectives can introduce additional questions, such as those identified in this chapter, that deepen the radical life extension conversation.

Notes

1 Sparks Therapeutics, Inc., 'Luxterna' (2019) retrieved from https://luxturna. com/#isi
2 www.hopkinsmedicine.org/stlm/history.html
3 https://papers.aarweb.org/pu/human-enhancement-and-transhumanism-unit

References

Agich, G. (2003). *Dependence and autonomy in old age: An ethical framework for long-term care.* Cambridge University Press. https://doi.org/10.1017/CBO9780511545801

Bagala, N. (2017). Will increased life spans be only for the rich? *Life Extension Advocacy Foundation.* www.leafscience.org/only-the-rich/

Beyret, E., Liao, H.-K., Yamamoto, M., Hernandez-Benitez, R., Fu, Y., Erikson, G., Reddy, P., & Izpisua Belmonte, J. C. (2019). Single-dose CRISPR-Cas9 therapy extends lifespan of mice with Hutchinson-Gilford progeria syndrome. *Nature Medicine, 25*(3), 419–422. https://doi.org/10.1038/s41591-019-0343-4

Bregman, L. (1999). *Beyond silence and denial – Death and dying reconsidered.* John Knox Press.

Browne, A., & Russell, J. S. (2016). Physician-assisted death in Canada. *Cambridge Quarterly of Healthcare Ethics, 25,* 37–383.

Burdett, M. (2015). The religion of technology: Transhumanism and the myth of progress. In C. Mercer & T. J. Trothen (Eds.), *Religion and transhumanism: The unknown future of human enhancement* (pp. 131–147). Praeger.

Burke, C., Wight, T., & Chenoweth, L. (2018). Supporting the spiritual needs of people with dementia in residential aged care. *Journal of Religion, Spirituality & Aging*, *30*(3), 234–250. https://doi.org/10.1080/15528030.2018.1434852

Chonody, J. M., & Teater, B. (2018). Aging and ageism: Cultural influences. In *Social work and practice with older adults: An actively aging framework for practice*. Sage Publications. http://doi.org/10.4135/9781506334271.n1

Cole-Turner, R. (2009). Extreme longevity research: A progressive Protestant perspective. In D. F. Maher & C. Mercer (Eds.), *Religion and the implications of radical life extension*. Palgrave MacMillan.

Collins, F. (2019, September 27). Gene therapy shows promise repairing brain tissue damaged by stroke. *National institutes of health: National institute on aging*. www.nia.nih.gov/news/gene-therapy-shows-promise-repairing-brain-tissue-damaged-stroke

Corey, G., Corey, M. S., Callanan, P., & Corey, C. (2015). *Issues and ethics in the helping professions* (9th ed.). Brooks/Cole/Cengage Learning.

de Grey, A. (2009). Radical life extension: Technological aspects. In D. F. Maher & C. Mercer (Eds.), *Religion and the implications of radical life extension* (pp. 13–24). Palgrave MacMillan.

Doehring, C. (2015). *The practice of pastoral care: A postmodern approach* (Revised and Expanded ed.). Westminster John Knox Press.

Donner, Y., Fortney, K., Calimport, S. R. G., Pfleger, K., Shah, M., & Betts-LaCroix, J. (2015). Great desire for extended life and health amongst the American public. *Frontiers in Genetics*, *6*, 353–353. https://doi.org/10.3389/fgene.2015.00353

Dreyfus, H. L., & Kelly, S. (2011). *All things shining: Reading the Western classics to find meaning in a secular age*. Free Press.

Ekerdt, D. J., Koss, C. S., Li, A., Münch, A., Lessenich, S., & Fung, H. H. (2017). Is longevity a value for older adults? *Journal of Aging Studies*, *43*, 46–52. https://doi.org/10.1016/j.jaging.2017.10.002

Feezell, R. (2013). *Sport, philosophy, and good lives*. University of Nebraska Press.

Fixed. (2013). *Fixed: The science/fiction of human enhancement*. A Making Change Media production; produced & directed by Regan Pretlow Brashear; co-producer, Jamie LeJeune, Blooming Grove, New York. New Day Films.

Foucault, M. (1988). *Technologies of the self*. University of Massachusetts Press.

Habermas, J. (1971). *Knowledge and human interests*. Beacon Press.

Hallberg, I. R. (2004). Death and dying from old people's point of view. A literature review. *Aging Clinical and Experimental Research*, *16*(2), 87–103. https://doi.org/10.1007/BF03324537

Hampton, M., Baydala, A., Bourassa, C., McKay-McNabb, K., Placsko, C., Goodwill, K., McKenna, B., McNabb, P., & Boekelder, R. (2010). Completing the circle: Elders speak about end-of-life care with aboriginal families in Canada. *Journal of Palliative Care*, *26*(1), 6–14. https://doi.org/10.1177/082585971002600103

Hanning, A. (2017). Talking about death in America: An anthropologist's view. *UNDARK*. https://undark.org/article/death-dying-america-anthropologist/

Hefner, P. (2009). The animal that aspires to be an angel: The challenge of transhumanism. *Dialog: A Journal of Theology*, *48*(2), 158–167. https://doi.org/10.1111/j.1540-6385.2009.00451.x

Hendry, M., Pasterfield, D., Lewis, R., Carter, B., Hodgson, D., & Wilkinson, C. (2013). Why do we want the right to die? A systematic review of the international literature on the views of patients, carers and the public on assisted dying. *Palliative Medicine*, *27*(1), 13–26. https://doi.org/10.1177/0269216312463623

Herzfeld, N. (2017). Must we die? Transhumanism, religion, and the fear of death. In T. J. Trothen & C. Mercer (Eds.), *Religion and human enhancement: Death, values, and morality* (pp. 285–300). Palgrave studies in the future of humanity and its successors series. Palgrave MacMillan.

Holman, W. (2013, April 12). Will Google's Ray Kurzweil live forever? *Wall Street Journal.* www.wsj.com/articles/SB10001424127887324504704578412581386515510

Holstein, M., Parks, J. A., & Waymack, M. H. (2011). *Ethics, aging, and society: The critical turn.* Springer Publishing Company.

Hopkins, P. D. (2015). A salvation paradox: *Saving* you versus saving *you.* In C. Mercer & T. J. Trothen (Eds.), *Religion and transhumanism: The unknown future of human enhancement* (pp. 71–82). Praeger.

Kim, G. J.-S., & Shaw, S. M. (2018). *Intersectional theology: An introductory guide.* Fortress Press.

Labrecque, C. A. (2015). Morphological freedom and the rebellion against human bodiliness: Notes from the Roman catholic tradition. In C. Mercer & T. Trothen (Eds.), *Religion and transhumanism: The unknown future of human enhancement* (pp. 303–313). Praeger.

Löckenhoff, C. E., De Fruyt, F., Terracciano, A., McCrae, R. R., De Bolle, M., Costa, P. T., Aguilar-Vafaie, M. E., Ahn, C.-K., Ahn, H.-N., Alcalay, L., Allik, J., Avdeyeva, T. V., Barbaranelli, C., Benet-Martinez, V., Blatný, M., Bratko, D., Brunner-Sciarra, M., Cain, T. R., Crawford, J. T., . . . & Yik, M. (2009). Perceptions of aging across 26 cultures and their culture-level associates. *Psychology and Aging, 24*(4), 941–954. https://doi.org/10.1037/a0016901

Maher, D. F., & Mercer, C. (2009). *Religions and the implications of radical life extension.* Palgrave MacMillan.

Marcuse, H. (1964). *One dimensional man: Studies in the ideology of advanced industrial society.* Beacon Press.

Mazanah, M., & Merriam, S. B. (2000). Aging and learning in a non-western culture: The case of Malaysia. *Adult education research conference.* Kansas State University Libraries. http://newprairiepress.org/aerc/2000/papers/57

McCracken, H., & Grossman, L. (2013). Can Google solve death? *Time Magazine.* https://content.time.com/time/subscriber/article/0,33009,2152422,00.html

Mercer, C., & Trothen, T. J. (2021). *Religion and the technological future: An introduction to Biohacking, A.I., and transhumanism.* Palgrave MacMillan.

Ory, M. G., Belza, B., & Smith, M. L. (2018). As life expectancies rise, so are expectations for healthy aging. *The Conversation.* https://theconversation.com/as-life-expectancies-rise-so-are-expectations-for-healthy-aging-102388

Pew Research Center. (2013). Religious leaders' views on radical life extension. *Pew Research Center.* Washington, DC. www.pewforum.org/2013/08/06/religious-leaders-views-on-radical-life-extension/

Powel, A. (2019). Longevity and anti-aging research: "Prime time for an impact on the globe". *The Harvard Gazette.* https://news.harvard.edu/gazette/story/2019/03/anti-aging-research-prime-time-for-an-impact-on-the-globe/

Purtill, C. (2019, October 4). Stop me if you've heard this one: A robot and a team of Irish scientists walk into a Senior Living Home. *TIME Magazine.* https://time.com/longform/senior-care-robot/

Seger, E. (2017, September 5). FDA approves first gene therapy for leukemia treatment: The how's, why's, promise, and peril. *The Science Distillery.*

https://sciencedistillery.wordpress.com/2017/09/05/fda-approves-first-gene-therapy-for-leukemia-treatment-the-hows-whys-promise-and-peril/

Sheridan, C. (2020). Go-ahead for first in-body CRISPR medicine testing. *Nature Biotechnology*. https://doi.org/10.1038/d41587-018-00003-2

Sherwin, S. (2012). A relational approach to autonomy in health care. In F. Baylis, J. Downie, B. Hoffmaster & S. Sherwin (Eds.), *Health care ethics in Canada* (3rd ed., pp. 242–257). Nelson.

Smith, J. (2019, July 10). Anti-aging gene therapy treats cardiovascular disease in mice. *Labiotech.eu*. www.labiotech.eu/medical/anti-aging-cardiovascular-disease/

Sparks Therapeutics, Inc. (2019). *Luxterna*. https://luxturna.com/#isi

Statistics Canada. (2019). *Canada's population estimates: Age and sex*. www150.stat-can.gc.ca/n1/en/daily-quotidien/190125/dq190125a-eng.pdf?st=q0L1DuLV

Trothen, T. J. (2017). Moral bioenhancement through an intersectional theo-ethical lens: Refocusing on divine image-bearing and interdependence. *Religions. Special Issue: Religion and the New Technologies*, *8*(5), 1–14. https://doi.org/10.3390/rel8050084

Vail, K., Juhl, J., Arndt, J., Vess, M., Routledge, C., & Rutjens, B. (2012). When death is good for life: Considering the positive trajectories of terror management. *Personality and Social Psychology Review*, *16*(4), 303–329. https://doi.org/10.1177/1088868312440046

Waldrop, D. P. (2011). Denying and defying death: The culture of dying in 21st century America. *The Gerontologist*, *51*(4), 571–576. https://doi.org/10.1093/geront/gnr076

World Health Organization. (2019). *Life expectancy*. www.who.int/gho/mortality_burden_disease/life_tables/situation_trends_text/en/

4 Assistive Technologies and Older Adults With Cognitive Problems

John Puxty

Introduction

The focus of this chapter is to identify how technology can promote greater independence and improve the quality of life of older adults with cognitive problems and in particular dementia.

Currently, dementia affects some 50 million people worldwide, and these numbers are expected to increase to 75 million in 2030 and 132 million by 2050 (WHO, 2012). Dementia is the fourth most common cause of death in developed countries (WHO, 2020) and many affected individuals die in long-term care institutions (Reyniers et al., 2015). Dementia is a chronic disease with enormous direct and indirect costs for the individual, caregivers, and society. In 2017, the World Health Organization declared it a public health priority and launched a public health plan (WHO, 2017). Dementia is recognized by policymakers and health providers as a condition of global significance and it is certainly relevant to the daily lives of Canadian families.

Under these circumstances, the care of dementia is multidimensional and constitutes a great challenge for caregivers and society (Wimo et al., 2011). To meet these complex needs, knowledge, skills, and strategies are required which span multiple disciplines in various sectors, ranging from home care, primary care, community and long-term care. In considering the use of assistive technologies within a dementia care plan, it is helpful to understand the spectrum and range of cognitive challenges that the individual and their caregivers may have to anticipate.

Normal Cognitive Changes With Aging

The normal aging process can bring subtle changes in cognitive abilities for some older adults (Harada et al., 2013). Committing new information to memory and recalling names and numbers can take longer. Autobiographical memory of life events and accumulated knowledge of learned facts and information – both types of *declarative memory* – may decline with age, whereas *procedural memories* like remembering how to ride a bike or tie a shoe remain

DOI: 10.4324/9781032617282-5

largely intact. *Working memory* – the ability to hold a piece of information in mind, such as a phone number, password, or the location of a parked car – is also susceptible to age-related changes. Other aspects of this kind of fluid intelligence, such as processing speed and problem-solving, may also decrease with age. And, certain aspects of attention can become more difficult as our brains age (Harada et al., 2013). For example, selective attention – our ability to tune out distractions and focus on a stimulus. Splitting our focus between two tasks – like holding a conversation while driving – can also become more challenging with age. This type of attention is called divided attention.

Generally, age-related changes in memory do not have functional, social or occupational significance and are readily adaptable by simple memory aides (making lists, repetition, use of visual associations, and saying things out aloud) reducing distractions and allowing more time for processing new information.

Mild Cognitive Impairment (MCI)

MCI is a neurological disorder which involves cognitive impairments beyond those expected based on an individual's age and education, but which are not significant enough to interfere with instrumental activities of daily living (Petersen, 2004). It may include both memory and non-memory impairments. Individuals with amnesic MCI have symptoms of memory loss in terms of failing to recall events and conversations, frequently misplacing items, missing appointments, and difficulty with recalling names. Non-amnestic MCI affects cognitive skills other than memory, including the ability to make sound decisions, judge the time or sequence of steps needed to complete a complex task or visual perception. It is characterized as an early indicator of cognitive impairment capable of further advancement to Alzheimer's disease (AD) or into another dementia with 10–15% progression yearly (Petersen, 2004). Individuals with MCI may particularly benefit from some of the technologies to support memory, function, safety, and way-finding described later.

Dementia

Dementia is a neurodegenerative chronic condition characterized by a progressive decline in a person's memory, thinking, learning skills, and ability to perform instrumental activities of daily life (IADLs) such as managing medications and finances, driving, shopping, preparing meals, use of public transportation, and care of household. Some of the commoner conditions seen are AD, dementia with Lewy bodies, vascular dementia, frontotemporal lobar degeneration, and Parkinson's disease.

The most common cognitive symptom especially in AD is memory loss. At the early onset and mild stage of the disease, short-term memory dysfunction is often the first complaint of the patients, manifesting as difficulty in learning new information. At later stages of the disease, substantial memory-recalling problems emerge (Gale, 2018). Other common associated cognitive issues are impacts on language, executive function, visuo-spatial perception, and mood.

Dementia is typically diagnosed at the time when cognitive impairments begin to affect the social and occupational functioning of the person although often by that time caregivers have been aware of concerns for at least a couple of years (Gale, 2018). As the illness progresses, impairments occur in visuo-constructional perceptual-motor functions, language functions, and social cognition (Hugo, 2014).

As an individual's dementia progresses, their ability to maintain independence and function change. In earlier stages, driving can be a concern along with troubles related to memory and executive function such as shopping and banking. In moderate stages, issues such as medication adherence, nutrition, falls, difficulties with way-finding and wandering become bigger concerns for families and caregivers. In the later stages, the ability for self-care and ADL's decline and patients may become dependent on others for functions such as eating, dressing, toileting, bathing, and mobility.

In conjunction with progressive cognitive deficits, dementia is often associated with behavioural and psychological symptoms such as agitation, depression, apathy, aggression, disinhibition, delusions, hallucinations, wandering, and sleep disruptions. This category of symptoms is sometimes also referred to as neuropsychiatric symptoms or responsive behaviours. They may be seen in all types of dementia although some patterns are associated more with certain types of dementia (Rockwood et al., 2015).

A diagnosis of dementia has a significant impact on caregivers and family members of people with dementia (PwD), who often bear the responsibility of caring for the individual as their health and functional independence deteriorates (Donelan et al., 2002). Individuals who provide unpaid and continuous assistance and have not been formally trained, such as spouses, children, or other family members, are referred to as informal caregivers, in contrast to formal caregivers, who offer paid services (Donelan et al., 2002). Furthermore, it is often the case that informal caregivers provide care to PwD in circumstances where formal health care does not reach because of healthcare systems' infrastructure, socioeconomic status, or cultural preferences, among others (Eales et al., 2015). Caregivers of PwDs spend more time on care than other caregivers (average of 13.6 versus 9.6 hour per week) and are at higher risk than other types of caregivers to feel overwhelmed and depressed. Commonly reported concerns of family caregivers are (i) the lack of safety in the home, (ii) lacking quality time for themselves, (iii) the absence of meaningful activities for people with dementia, and (iv) difficulties experienced with time orientation.

In the lack of a cure for dementia, the focus of management is towards early identification, seeking to postpone its onset and rate of progress, attempting to compensate for cognitive deficits, promote socialization, and maintain function while reducing stress on caregivers. Early detection of the disease is of relevance due to the increased possibilities for early initiation of treatment, and other forms of disease management interventions.

Assistive Technologies and Dementia

Significant research and development efforts have been emerging in the last decade into the design and development of assistive technologies for the elderly, in general, and the dementia patients in particular. A wide variety of Smart-Health (s-Health) technologies are being developed to help older adults, chronic illness patients, and their informal caregivers at home and are showing promising results (Chouvarda et al., 2015; Darkins et al., 2008). The use of s-Health technologies for dementia is a constantly evolving field that includes assisted living technology, ambient-assisted living technologies and smart homes, among other devices and systems. Cahill and colleagues (2007) proposed that s-Health technologies fall into four main categories, namely, (1) those used to promote safety, (2) those that foster communication and address memory loss problems, (3) those that provide multisensory stimulation, and (4) those that act as memory enhancers.

The remainder of this chapter will focus on some of the relevant developments in technology and product development and propose strategies by which they may be integrated into the following: early diagnosis and assessment; modifying disease progress and its impact; aiding memory; maintaining functional abilities; promoting safety and independence; socialization and recreation; and supporting the caregiver and relieving stress.

Early Diagnosis and Assessment

Probably one of the most developed and researched uses of technology in dementia is for conducting cognitive assessments. These products are aimed primarily at healthcare professionals offering cognitive assessments, and organizations, particularly pharmaceutical companies, conducting research trials. One of the earliest technology-based cognitive assessment batteries – Cambridge Neuropsychological Test Automated Battery (CANTAB) (Barnett et al., 2015) – was developed in the late 1980s and early 1990s using touchscreen technology. According to the developers at the University of Cambridge:

> Cambridge Neuropsychological Test Automated Battery (CANTAB) includes highly sensitive, precise and objective measures of cognitive function, correlated to neural networks. CANTAB tests have demonstrated sensitivity to detecting changes in neuropsychological performance and include tests of working memory, learning and executive function; visual, verbal and episodic memory; attention, information processing and reaction time; social and emotion recognition, decision making and response control.[1]

CANTAB is now marketed worldwide through Cambridge Cognition as a tool for running drug and other large-scale trials.

The advent of smartphones, tablets, smartwatches, and other wearable devices has created opportunities for new mobile assessments (Chinner et al., 2018; Pillai & Bonner-Jackson, 2015). There are also websites such as Cogniciti where people concerned about their memory can complete a short online test to see if they should consult their doctor. In addition, the potential of VR for assessing people with dementia is also being explored with early projects such as virtual navigation (Cushman et al., 2008) and VIRTUALKITCHEN (Allain et al., 2014) demonstrating possible impacts for some users.

Rehabilitation and Cognitive Training

In a study with 21 participants of "Kitchen and cooking", a serious game developed for older adults with cognitive impairment demonstrated improved concentration but there was no investigation of transference to actual cooking tasks (Manera et al., 2015).

The possibility of using virtual reality and augmented reality technologies to deliver cognitive rehabilitation is promising. García-Betances and colleagues (2015) produced a review and guidelines (García-Betances, 2015) for developing cognitive rehabilitation and training using VR functionality. A systematic review (Moreno et al., 2019) of the use of virtual reality for cognitive rehabilitation in individuals with neurocognitive disorders suggested that it improved cognition in areas such as memory, dual tasking and visual attention, and secondarily acted on psychological functions such as reduction of anxiety, higher levels of wellbeing, and increased use of coping strategies.

Although there are some promising results for cognitive rehabilitation, the evidence currently available does not support recommending "brain training" through various commercially available apps or devices. Lumosity, for example, was fined in 2016 by the US Federal Trade Commission (FTC) for "deceptive advertising" regarding its claims to "delay cognitive impairment". Another app, MindMate, advertises "*get fitter, improve your brain health and stay independent for as long as possible*". Some of the contents of this app (games, physical activity, and nutrition) are based on evidence from research studies, particularly the FINGER[2] study which explored the impact of a multi-domain intervention on the cognitive function of older adults are risk of dementia. However, the app is independent of the FINGER researchers and there is not enough peer-reviewed research published to support the efficacy of the app itself.

Memory Aids

There are a number of different devices available for setting reminders, which can include a voice recording of the individual or family member. Types of prompts and reminders include the following:

Devices that detect motion: These use a sensor or pressure mat and play a pre-recorded voice when there is movement. For example, to play a message when you walk out of the kitchen to remind you to turn off the stove.

Devices that play set reminders: These play messages at certain times. For example, recording a message reminding to take medication. Using calendar apps such as Google Calendar can be helpful when caregivers are overloaded with tasks to remember or when trying to coordinate a network of care. Calendars can be set to generate automated reminders – whether that is several times a day or once a year – and can be used for keeping track of medication schedules, doctor appointments, or when test results are due. The calendar can be shared, too, allowing more than one person to set reminders, and "invite" others to see the calendar, allowing multiple caregivers to be aware of forthcoming appointments and events.

Android Master is an early example of one such app for Android devices which lets you record your voice to play for a reminder to take pills, drink water, or turn off the lights, for example. The app can also record the user's reaction, which could be useful for caregivers to help track how their loved one is doing on a regular basis.

Medication aids: There are a lot of different aids that assist in taking medication at the right time. These include simple pill boxes (often known as dosette boxes) – with separate compartments for days of the week and times of day – or more sophisticated automatic pill dispensers that set off an alarm and the right compartment opens so that the individual can access the correct pills for the time slot. Some devices can be set so the alarm goes off until the pills are removed. This can also include alerting friends or family if the medication hasn't been taken, or if there's a problem with the device (e.g., the battery is low or it needs refilling).

Locator devices: A locator device can be used to find common misplaced things such as keys or a wallet. A small electronic tag is attached to each item. Locator devices can work in different ways. In some systems, if an item gets lost, pressing a button on a dedicated locator device will activate the tag with a beeping noise, a flashing light, or a combination of both.

Another option is to attach a small tile to each item and link them to a smartphone using an app. The location of the item can then be shown on the phone's map app. Some apps will store the last place where the phone "saw" the tile. Jiobit is one such example, which, while originally designed to keep track of kids, can also be a powerful way to keep tabs on an older adult who might wander off. There are several ways to securely attach it so it's not easily removed. One helpful feature: You can set a "geofence" to alert you when the person leaves the designated "trusted place". Jiobit even learns the person's usual movements and alerts you if they go somewhere else.

Socialization and Recreation

Communication and Socialization

Technology-based support for communication and social interaction has also long been a focus of investigation. For example, Astell in 2008 described a Computer Interactive Reminiscing and Conversation Aid (CIRCA) which includes a touchscreen-based interactive, multimedia conversation support containing generic contents, developed in partnership with people with dementia and caregivers. In 2015, Ekström, Ferm, and Samuelsson created a personalized version of CIRCA for an individual with young onset dementia and reported a positive impact on her communication.

In terms of mainstream technology, people with dementia often initially continue to use email, cell phones, texts, and apps such as Zoom, Skype, FaceTime, and Google Hangout if they used them before. Zoom and its predecessor Skype have been popular in long-term care as a means of connecting residents with family. There are also dementia-specific commercial products, such as simple cell phones [e.g., Memory Picture Phone and Dial-Less Phone (Canada), Doro (UK), and the KISA phone (Australia)].

Fun and Games

Another important application of technology is to support people with dementia to engage with and enjoy leisure activities. Just like the rest of the population, people with dementia seek meaningful and enjoyable activities. Games can provide this satisfaction but despite the millions of games in online stores, very few are dementia-friendly, for example, accessible for people with dementia. To address this the AcToDementia[3] (Accessible Touchscreen Apps for People Living with Dementia), website is a resource containing reviews of games in different categories (e.g., card games and art games), that have been identified for their dementia-friendly features.

In addition to apps, game systems are popular mainstream devices that can be enjoyed by people with dementia as a group activity or something to play with their grandchildren. Dove and Astell (2019), for example, set up an Xbox Kinect bowling group. Based on their experience, Astell and colleagues (2018) produced system development guidelines for other developers and researchers interested in utilizing motion-based technologies for dementia.

Other activities developed specifically for people with dementia include viewing art on a tablet (Tyack et al., 2017), creating art on touchscreen devices (Leuty et al., 2013), digital storytelling delivered on an app (Critten & Kucirkova, 2019), and House of Memories[4] (UK), a museum-led dementia awareness program using an app to explore historical artefacts.

Maintaining Function, Safety, and Independence

Smart Homes

Delivering interventions to people with dementia directly where they live in response to changes detected in the surroundings has been another popular focus of technology research and product development. Emphasizing the potential for maintaining people with dementia at home and delivering care remotely, numerous products and systems utilizing sensors and instrumented devices have been developed.

This can be as simple as using virtual assistants (such as those by Amazon or Google or ElliQ) that allow you to give voice commands or ask questions, which they then carry out or answer. This can range from asking what the weather is like, to creating an entire "smart home" system which plays music, controls the lights, and adjusts the central heating (although additional equipment would be needed for these). These devices work using "artificial intelligence" which means that over time they become more useful as they "learn" to recognize a voice and personalize the responses. They can be useful for lots of different purposes such as adding a home alarm system that will "listen" for sounds like glass breaking and can alert you remotely. They can also be programmed to provide reminders about appointments or when to take medication or make phone calls. When set up and programmed by a caregiver, these devices can provide a sense of control and comfort for the person with early to mild dementia and help reduce their feelings of social isolation and boredom.

Additionally, individual items such as bed occupancy sensors, floor mat sensors, door opening alerts, motion detection, and activity monitors can be purchased online for individuals and organizations to establish their own monitoring systems. In addition to custom and off-the-shelf technologies, a number of websites offer advice on creating a "dementia-friendly home". As with the GPS devices, these products are largely purchased by care providers (formal and informal) although some, such as the My Intelligent Home (Miihome) project (UK), are now being co-created with people who have dementia to provide ambient support to maintain their activities of daily living (Caliskanelli et al., 2019)

Research is ongoing in integrating a number of devices include SmartCondo™ and smart apartment (Canada), the Gloucester Smart Home (Orpwood et al., 2004) and Deptford smart flat (Orpwood et al., 2004; UK), and Dem@ Care and DOMUS smart apartment (France). In the United Kingdom, the 2016–2018 technology Integrated Health Management (TIHM) project is a joint healthcare/academic/industry Internet of Things project utilizing existing devices to monitor the health of people with dementia at home. Commercially available smart home systems include CareLink Advantage (Canada), CareSensus (a partnership between Philips and Cordaan, a Dutch care provider), Just Checking and Canary Care (UK), and Abilia (Europe).

Robots

Research into robotics generally has gathered pace over recent years. In health care for older adults, efforts fall into several areas including robots as direct caregivers, assistants, companions, and facilitators of social interaction in older adults both with (Gerłowska et al., 2020) and without dementia (Van Patten et al., 2020).

The subcategory of robots that serve to provide social facilitation and companionship to users with dementia is socially assistive robots (SARs).

Attempts to develop SARs for interaction with dementia patients are not uncommon. The so-called social companionship robots have taken the form of relatively simple pseudo-animal robots made of metal or with synthetic fur, such as NeCoRo, AIBO, and Paro, which represent a cat, dog, and baby harp seal, respectively, and have been implemented in older adult care-homes (Mordoch et al., 2013). A 2004 study utilizing NeCoRo, a robotic cat featuring synthetic fur, lifelike behaviours, and an ability to respond to user touch (Libin & Libin, 2003), to residents of a nursing home for dementia patients, observed a decrease in general agitation. One of the more successful implementations of an animal-like SAR is Paro, the robotic baby harp seal. Paro is equipped with synthetic fur, and a variety of sensors that allow its behaviour to change based on user input. A 2013 study comparing the effects of Paro to those of a resident dog presented Paro to care-home residents twice a week over the course of 12 weeks. Like the dog, the robot significantly decreased loneliness in residents, and the novelty of the device stimulated conversation between residents more than the resident dog (Robinson et al., 2013). Several other studies, however, have suggested that although there can be benefits to the use of these robot pets with dementia patients, their value is primarily for entertainment and they should not be presented as if they are real (e.g., Scerri et al., 2021; Koh et al., 2021). In addition, healthy older adults not suffering from dementia tend to prefer living animals rather than robots.

Another area of considerable interest in applying robotics to dementia care comes in the form of cognitive-assistive robots and technologies that aid users in performing activities of daily living. Such devices typically have roles in helping patients to maintain a schedule and remember certain tasks. More complicated models use computer vision to determine what the user is trying to do, and prompt them to perform the task correctly. One example is the "COACH" system that was designed to assist dementia patients with handwashing. The system is capable of recognizing handwashing steps, as seen through a camera, and prompts the user with audio and shows video demonstrations, as necessary. The system increased the ability of most subjects to complete handwashing steps independently and reduced the need for caregiver intervention (Mihailidis et al., 2008) A robot prototyped in 2013 was developed similarly to identify steps in the process of making tea and intervene as needed. Though most of the participants in this study had the cognitive capacity to complete the task themselves, the subjects and their caregivers reported interest in the robot, noting that it was useful, and would be nice to have at a later stage of the subject's disease (Begum et al., 2013).

Nejat and colleagues created Brian, a humanoid robot developed to support people living with dementia in long-term care facilities at mealtimes. Brian's creators have also developed Casper (McColl & Nejat, 2013), a prototype robot to prompt people through the steps of meal preparation, and Tangy (McColl & Nejat, 2013) a non-humanoid robot to support bingo in care homes.

Other developments have utilized telepresence robots which are basically a video conferencing system controlled by a remote user, for example, rather than appearing on a fixed desktop monitor or screen, the person speaking/viewing (family member or caregiver) can move the robot around the environment of the individual. Early models of telepresence robots on the consumer market include Giraff, Anybots® (QB), Beampro™, VGO, PadBot, Double Robotics, and MantaroBot (Kristoffersson et al., 2013), with new products under development. One of these, Giraff, has been developed and used in a number of European research projects focused on supporting older adults at home by combining the robot with a network of sensors (Coradeschi et al., 2013). A 2019 study noted that family carers of PwD in LTC reported a feeling of presence and connectedness when talking to their family member via the telepresence robots (Moyle et al., 2020). They reported the robots as helping to enhance longer conversations and social connection with their family member.

Currently, the bulk of robot research and testing continues to be focused on dementia care as well as combatting loneliness, social isolation, and prompting people with daily tasks. There is evidence of broad acceptability both by PwD and caregivers (Wang et al., 2017); however, there remains much work to be done before these can be deployed at scale.

Supporting Care and Reducing Caregiver Stress

Monitoring and Tracking

Technology in various forms has also been used to monitor people with dementia both at home and outside during various activities. Much of this monitoring has arisen in response to concerns from caregivers about the safety and security of people with dementia, for instance, during activities such as cooking or when leaving home unaccompanied. This has given rise to one of the more controversial uses of technology in dementia (Landau, 2012), namely the application of electronic tagging and global positioning systems (GPSs) as responses to people with dementia going out unaccompanied.

Back in 2005, Miskelley tested the feasibility of using specific electronic tracking devices to locate people who have dementia via a GPS-enabled cell phone. Since then, numerous devices have emerged and are commercially available online. These include wearables (e.g., GPS watch), attachables (GPS devices for clothing, belts, etc.), insertables (GPS insoles), and portable GPS trackers (to go in bags, pockets).

Multiple companies now exist specializing in these products with prices ranging from affordable devices to those that cost hundreds or even thousands of dollars for a system of several connected devices and services. The majority of these are aimed at family caregivers or care organizations to monitor the people they care for. The evidence base for these products relates to the efficiency and reliability of the GPS technology and success in locating individuals.

Caregiver Education

For formal caregivers, a range of web-based training interventions have been developed. The CARES program developed for nursing assistants was shown to improve new information and skills and reduce stress relating to caregiving (Hobday et al., 2010). Technology has also been applied to creating integrated care packages for people with dementia, such as the intervention-management-system developed by Eichler and colleagues to suggest recommendations to GPs (Eichler et al., 2014).

Communication

Technology-based support for communication and social interaction has also long been a focus of investigation. For example, CIRCA, described by Astell in 2008, which consists of a touchscreen-based interactive, multimedia conversation support containing generic contents, developed in partnership with people with dementia and caregivers. In 2015, Ekström, Ferm and Samuelsson created a personalized version of CIRCA for a woman with young onset dementia and reported a positive impact on her communication. While newly developed communication supports are compelling, many people with dementia can continue to use email, cell phones, texts, and communication apps if they used them before.

Caregiving

Maresova and colleagues (2018) noted that a common focus of technology use in older adults with AD was monitoring the PwD or improving the working conditions or comfort levels of the caregiver. Assistive technologies have a role in supporting informal caregivers of PwD for situations often associated with informal caregiving, such as symptoms of depression, stress and anxiety, or caring burden (Torkamani et al., 2014). A survey of 72 family caregivers identified the features of devices which they perceived as being most useful: prior familiarity with the technology; intuitiveness; ease of use; and ability to simplify activities and prevent accidents, with safety often given priority over the privacy and autonomy of their relatives with dementia (Mao et al., 2015).

In care services, the use of technology is expanding rapidly to encompass a wide range of activities, which demand a technology-enabled workforce. For example, Hammond Care[5] uses technology to support delivery of care through smart systems in the cottages where their residents live. These systems include sensors for monitoring routines, addressing issues (e.g., falls), silent nurse call system, and environmental monitoring. They also utilize PainChek™, an app to assess pain in people with dementia, which uses artificial intelligence and smartphone technology to visually analyse facial expressions, assess pain levels in real time, and update cloud-based medical records. Hammond Care is also a partner in developing the Virtual Reality-Empathy Platform (VR-EP), a software that enables architects, designers, and builders to explore potential environments as if they were a person with dementia.

Uptake of Technology

A systematic review by Holthe in 2018 on the use of technology in community-dwelling older adults with mild MCI or dementia identified 29 peer-reviewed studies published between 2007 and 2017 which spanned four main domains: safe walking (indoors and outdoors), technologies for enhancing safe living, improvement in ADLs, and finally technologies for entertainment and leisure. They noted that very few studies reported perceptions of the acceptability and usability of the technologies or on the consequences of technology on the quality of life and occupational performance. When reported, the usability and acceptability of technologies often depended on whether the technology addressed an individual's self-perceived need without intruding upon the individual's character or identity.

Evans et al. (2015) also found that many assistive technology systems had a limited place in real-life cases because of their low acceptance and adoption, often relating this to privacy, usability, and cost issues. Although the use of Internet and mobile devices by older adults increases yearly, there is still variable uptake of health technologies. Sensory (visual, auditory, touch perception, mobility, and balance) and cognition (memory, attention, and spatial cognition) changes with aging may make use of new technologies difficult (Mao et al., 2015). Social and cultural factors may also affect interest and comfort with devices that the senior interacts with directly. Costs of these technologies are decreasing but can still represent a practical or psychological barrier.

Contrary to common belief, however, older adults do display positive attitudes towards technology, suggesting that uptake will increase, particularly, if perceived benefits start to increase (Smith, 2013). If new technologies take the cognitive, sensory, and emotional needs of older adults into account, it is expected that adoption will increase, especially as the "next generation" of older adults will be much more tech-savvy. In addition, current research is investigating how to personalize existing technologies to better fit users' needs and work with their personality traits. Exposure and support are also important in gaining acceptance.

The advent and rapid uptake of smartphones and tablets in the last 10 years has opened up access to personal computing to many new audiences and created increasing interest in how such devices can be used to empower people. Similarly, growing awareness and availability of emerging technologies such as robots, virtual reality (VR), smart home systems, and autonomous (e.g., driverless) vehicles are causing an explosion of interest in how they can improve wellbeing, including for those living with dementia. Although it has only recently gained mainstream attention, research applying technology to dementia has been taking place alongside biomedical research for many decades (Maresova et al., 2018). However, technology development has received comparatively little funding, resulting in much research that is limited to pilot or feasibility studies. Consequently, the amount and range of evidence-based technological interventions for dementia are small but growing.

Summary

While there are currently no disease-modifying drug therapies for any dementia subtypes and little drug discovery research into the less common ones, there is huge potential for technology, in the forms of devices, applications and services, to assess and optimize functioning of people to live with dementia. In addition, technology can benefit families caring for a relative with dementia through dedicated devices and services, plus support through online forums and education about dementia. Technology can also support service providers through a digitally enabled workforce, assessment and monitoring functions, and provision of interventions.

While research into technology for dementia has been underway for many decades and has already made great progress in some areas, there are still many gaps (Lorenz et al., 2019; Meiland et al., 2017; Boots et al., 2014). Most notable is the relatively small number of products aimed at supporting individuals who have dementia to address their cognitive challenges and maintain their daily and leisure activities.

By far, the bulk of research and commercial products have targeted family and organizational care providers plus research and pharmaceutical organizations conducting cognitive assessments. This may reflect perceptions of who the intended or likely consumers of the research and products are.

There is also a real issue about who should pay for and support the purchase, deployment, and maintenance of technology for people with dementia. For example, a smartphone provides telephone calling, text, email and video access to family, and services to combat social isolation, calendars for scheduling and reminding which can be shared with caregivers, GPS for monitoring, maps, and a compass to support navigation, games for cognitive stimulation and recreation, but it is unlikely at the present time that a healthcare provider or insurance company would pay for a phone and the data package for a person with dementia. Necessities for the future of this field will include increased awareness among healthcare providers of available technologies and functionality, engagement by companies with people with dementia or care providers and realistic proposals for funding the solutions to keep people with dementia well at home for as long as possible.

Notes

1 www.cambridgecognition.com/cantab
2 www.alz.org/wwfingers/overview.asp
3 www.actodementia.com
4 https://houseofmemories.co.uk/app
5 www.hammond.com.au/

References

Allain, P., Foloppe, D. A., Besnard, J., Yamaguchi, T., Etcharry-Bouyx, F., Le Gall, D., Nolin, P., & Richard, P. (2014). Detecting everyday action deficits in Alzheimer's disease using a non-immersive virtual reality kitchen. *Journal of the International Neuropsychological Society, 20*(5), 468–477. https://doi.org/10.1017/S1355617714000344

Astell, A. J., Smith, S. K., Potter, S., & Preston-Jones, E. (2018). Computer interactive reminiscence and conversation aid groups – Delivering cognitive stimulation with technology. *Alzheimer's & Dementia: Translational Research & Clinical Interventions, 4*(1), 481–487. https://doi.org/10.1016/j.trci.2018.08.003

Barnett, J. H., Blackwell, A. D., Sahakian, B. J., & Robbins, T. W. (2015). The paired associates learning (PAL) test: 30 years of CANTAB translational neuroscience from laboratory to bedside in dementia research. In T. W. Robbins & B. J. Sahakian (Eds.), *Translational neuropsychopharmacology. Current topics in behavioral neurosciences.* Springer. https://doi.org/10.1007/7854_2015_5001

Begum, M., Wang, R., Huq, R., & Mihailidis, A. (2013). Performance of daily activities by older adults with dementia: The role of an assistive robot. *IEEE . . . International conference on rehabilitation robotics: [Proceedings], 2013*, 6650405. https://doi.org/10.1109/ICORR.2013.6650405

Boots, L. M., de Vugt, M. E., van Knippenberg, R. J., Kempen, G. I., & Verhey, F. R. (2014). A systematic review of Internet-based supportive interventions for caregivers of patients with dementia. *International Journal of Geriatric Psychiatry, 29*(4), 331–344. https://doi.org/10.1002/gps.4016

Cahill, S., Begley, E., Faulkner, J. P., & Hagen, I. H. (2007). "It gives me a sense of independence" findings from Ireland on the use and usefulness of assistive technology for people with dementia. *Technology and Disability, 19*, 133–142. http://doi.org/10.3233/TAD-2007-192-310

Caliskanelli, I., Nefti-Meziani, S., Drake, J., & Hodgson, A. (2019). My intelligent home (MiiHome) project. In T. Ahram & C. Falcão (Eds.), *Advances in usability, user experience and assistive technology. Advances in intelligent systems and computing* (Vol. 794). Springer. https://doi.org/10.1007/978-3-319-94947-5_77

Chinner, A., Blane, J., Lancaster, C., Hinds, C., & Koychev, I. (2018). Digital technologies for the assessment of cognition: A clinical review. *Evidence-Based Mental Health, 21*(2), 67–71. https://doi.org/10.1136/eb-2018-102890

Chouvarda, I. G., Goulis, D. G., Lambrinoudaki, I., & Maglaveras, N. (2015). Connected health and integrated care: Toward new models for chronic disease management. *Maturitas, 82*(1), 22–27. https://doi.org/10.1016/j.maturitas.2015.03.015

Coradeschi, S., Cesta, A., Cortellessa, G., Coraci, L., Galindo, C., Gonzalez, J., Karlsson, L., Forsberg, A., Frennert, S., Furfari, F., Loutfi, A., Orlandini, A., Palumbo, F., Pecora, F., von Rump, S., Štimec, A., Ullberg, J., & Ötslund, B. (2013). GiraffPlus: A system for monitoring activities and physiological parameters and promoting social interaction for elderly. *Human-Computer Systems Interaction: Backgrounds and Applications, 3*, 261–271. https://doi.org/10.1007/978-3-319-08491-6_22

Critten, V., & Kucirkova, N. (2019). "It brings it all back, all those good times; it makes me go close to tears". Creating digital personalised stories with people who have dementia. *Dementia*, *18*, 864–881. https://doi.org/10.1177/1471301217691162

Cushman, L. A., Stein, K., & Duffy, C. J. (2008). Detecting navigational deficits in cognitive aging and Alzheimer disease using virtual reality. *Neurology*, *71*(12), 888–895. https://doi.org/10.1212/01.wnl.0000326262.67613.fe

Darkins, A., Ryan, P., Kobb, R., Foster, L., Edmonson, E., Wakefield, B., & Lancaster, A. E. (2008). Care coordination/home telehealth: The systematic implementation of health informatics, home telehealth, and disease management to support the care of veteran patients with chronic conditions. *Telemedicine Journal and E-health*, *14*(10), 1118–1126. https://doi.org/10.1089/tmj.2008.0021

Donelan, K., Hill, C. A., Hoffman, C., Scoles, K., Feldman, P. H., Levine, C., & Gould, D. (2002). Challenged to care: Informal caregivers in a changing health system. *Health Affairs*, *21*(4), 222–231. https://doi.org/10.1377/hlthaff.21.4.222

Dove, E., & Astell, A. J. (2019). Kinect project: People with dementia or mild cognitive impairment learning to play group motion-based games. *Alzheimer's & Dementia: Translational Research & Clinical Interventions*, *5*, 475–482. https://doi.org/10.1016/j.trci.2019.07.008

Eales, J., Kim, C., & Fast, J. (2015). A snapshot of Canadians caring for persons with dementia: The toll it takes. *Research on aging, policies, and practice*. https://rapp.ualberta.ca/Portals/116/Documents/FactSheets/2015-10 Dementia Caregivers in Canada.pdf

Eichler, T., Thyrian, J., Fredrich, D., Köhler, L., Wucherer, D., Michalowsky, B., Dreier, A., & Hoffmann, W. (2014). The benefits of implementing a computerized Intervention-Management-System (IMS) on delivering integrated dementia care in the primary care setting. *International Psychogeriatrics*, *26*(8), 1377–1385. https://doi.org/10.1017/S1041610214000830

Ekström, A., Ferm, U., & Samuelsson, C. (2015). Digital communication support and Alzheimer's disease. *Dementia*, *6*(16), 711–731. https://doi.org/10.1177/1471301215615456

Evans, J., Brown, M. A., Coughlan, T., Lawson, G., & Craven, M. P. (2015). A systematic review of dementia focused assistive technology In M. Kurosu (Ed.), *Human-computer interaction: Interaction technologies*. Lecture notes in computer science series, 9170 (pp. 406–417). https://doi.org/10.1007/978-3-319-20916-6_38

Gale, S. A., Acar, D., & Daffner, K. R. (2018). Dementia. *American Journal of Medicine*, *131*(10), 1161–1169. https://doi.org/10.1016/j.amjmed.2018.01.022

García-Betances, R. I., Arredondo Waldmeyer, M. T., Fico, G., & Cabrera-Umpiérrez, M. F. (2015). A succinct overview of virtual reality technology use in Alzheimer's disease. *Frontiers in Aging Neuroscience*, *7*(80). https://doi.org/10.3389/fnagi.2015.00080

García-Betances, R. I., Jiménez-Mixco, V., Arredondo, M. T., & Cabrera-Umpiérrez, M. F. (2015). Using virtual reality for cognitive training of the elderly. *American Journal of Alzheimer's Disease and other Dementias*, *30*(1), 49–54. https://doi.org/10.1177/1533317514545866

Gerłowska, J., Furtak-Niczyporuk, M., & Rejdak, K. (2020). Robotic assistance for people with dementia: A viable option for the future? *Expert Review of Medical Devices, 17*(6), 507–518. https://doi.org/10.1080/17434440.2020.1770592

Gillis, C., Mirzaei, F., Potashman, M., Ikram, M. A., & Maserejian, N. (2019). The incidence of mild cognitive impairment: A systematic review and data synthesis. *Alzheimer's & Dementia: Diagnosis, Assessment & Disease Monitoring, 11*, 248–256. https://doi.org/10.1016/j.dadm.2019.01.004

Harada, C. N., Natelson Love, M. C., & Triebel, K. L. (2013). Normal cognitive aging. *Clinics in Geriatric Medicine, 29*(4), 737–752. https://doi.org/10.1016/j.cger.2013.07.002

Hobday, J. V., Savik, K., Smith, S., & Gaugler, J. E. (2010). Feasibility of Internet training for care staff of residents with dementia: The CARES program. *Journal of Gerontological Nursing, 36*(4), 13–21. https://doi.org/10.3928/00989134-20100302-01

Holthe, T., Halvorsrud, L., Karterud, D., Hoel, K. A., & Lund, A. (2018). Usability and acceptability of technology for community-dwelling older adults with mild cognitive impairment and dementia: A systematic literature review. *Clinical Interventions in Aging, 13*, 863–886. https://doi.org/10.2147/CIA.S154717

Hugo, J., & Ganguli, M. (2014). Dementia and cognitive impairment: Epidemiology, diagnosis, and treatment. *Clinics in Geriatric Medicine, 30*(3), 421–442. https://doi.org/10.1016/j.cger.2014.04.001

Koh, W. Q., Ang, F., & Casey, D. (2021). Impacts of low-cost robotic pets for older adults and people with dementia: Scoping review. *JMIR Rehabilitation and Assistive Technologies, 8*(1), e25340. https://doi.org/10.2196/25340

Kristoffersson, A., Coradeschi, S., & Loutfi, A. (2013). A review of mobile robotic telepresence. *Advances in Human-Computer Interaction*, 902316. https://doi.org/10.1155/2013/902316

Landau, R., & Werner, S. (2012). Ethical aspects of using GPS for tracking people with dementia: Recommendations for practice. *International Psychogeriatrics, 24*(3), 358–366. https://doi.org/10.1017/S1041610211001888

Leuty, V., Boger, J., Young, L., Hoey, J., & Mihailidis, A. (2013). Engaging older adults with dementia in creative occupations using artificially intelligent assistive technology. *Assistive Technology: The Official Journal of RESNA, 25*(2), 72–79. https://doi.org/10.1080/10400435.2012.715113

Libin, E., & Libin, A. (2003). New diagnostic tool for robotic psychology and robotherapy studies. *Cyberpsychology & Behavior: The Impact of the Internet, Multimedia and Virtual Reality on Behavior and Society, 6*(4), 369–374.

Lorenz, K., Freddolino, P. P., Comas-Herrera, A., Knapp, M., & Damant, J. (2019). Technology-based tools and services for people with dementia and carers: Mapping technology onto the dementia care pathway. *Dementia, 18*(2), 725–741. https://doi.org/10.1177/1471301217691617

Manera, V., Petit, P. D., Derreumaux, A., Orvieto, I., Romagnoli, M., Lyttle, G., David, R., & Robert, P. H. (2015). "Kitchen and cooking," a serious game for mild cognitive impairment and Alzheimer's disease: A pilot study. *Frontiers in Aging Neuroscience, 7*, 24. https://doi.org/10.3389/fnagi.2015.00024

Mao, H. F., Chang, L. H., Yao, G., Chen, W. Y., & Huang, W. N. (2015). Indicators of perceived useful dementia care assistive technology: Caregivers' perspectives. *Geriatrics & Gerontology International*, *15*(8), 1049–1057. https://doi.org/10.1111/ggi.12398

Maresova, P., Tomsone, S., Lameski, P., Madureira, J., Mendes, A., Zdravevski, E., Chorbev, I., Trajkovik, V., Ellen, M., & Rodile, K. (2018). Technological solutions for older people with Alzheimer's disease: Review. *Current Alzheimer Research*, *15*(10), 975–983. https://doi.org/10.2174/1567205015666618042 7124547

McColl, D., & G. Nejat, G. (2013). Meal-time with a socially assistive robot and older adults at a long-term care facility. *Journal of Human-Robot Interaction*, *2*(1), 152–171.

Meiland, F., Innes, A., Mountain, G., Robinson, L., van der Roest, H., García-Casal, J. A., Gove, D., Thyrian, J. R., Evans, S., Dröes, R. M., Kelly, F., Kurz, A., Casey, D., Szcześniak, D., Dening, T., Craven, M. P., Span, M., Felzmann, H., Tsolaki, M., & Franco-Martin, M. (2017). Technologies to support community-dwelling persons with dementia: A position paper on issues regarding development, usability, effectiveness and cost-effectiveness, deployment, and ethics. *JMIR Rehabilitation and Assistive Technologies*, *4*(1), e1. https://doi.org/10.2196/rehab.6376

Mihailidis, A., Boger, J., Craig, T., & Hoey, J. (2008). The COACH prompting system to assist older adults with dementia through handwashing: An efficacy study. *BMC Geriatrics*, *8*, 28–28. https://doi.org/10.1186/1471-2318-8-28

Mordoch, E., Osterreicher, A., Guse, L., Roger, K., & Thompson, G. (2013). Use of social commitment robots in the care of elderly people with dementia: A literature review. *Maturitas*, *74*, 14–20.

Moreno, A., Wall, K. J., Thangavelu, K., Craven, L., Ward, E., & Dissanayaka, N. N. (2019). A systematic review of the use of virtual reality and its effects on cognition in individuals with neurocognitive disorders. *Alzheimer's & Dementia*, *5*, 834–850. https://doi.org/10.1016/j.trci.2019.09.016

Moyle, W., Jones, C., & Sung, B. (2020). Telepresence robots: Encouraging interactive communication between family carers and people with dementia. *Australasian Journal on Ageing*, *39*, e127–e133.

Orpwood, R., Gibbs, C., Adlam, T., Faulkner, R., & Meegahawatte, D. (2004). *The Gloucester smart house for people with dementia – User-interface aspects*. https://doi.org/10.1007/978-0-85729-372-5_24.

Petersen, R. C. (2004). Mild cognitive impairment as a diagnostic entity. *Journal of Internal Medicine*, *256*(3), 183–194. https://doi.org/10.1111/j.1365-2796.2004.01388.x

Pillai, J. A., & Bonner-Jackson, A. (2015). Review of information and communication technology devices for monitoring functional and cognitive decline in Alzheimer's disease clinical trials. *Journal of Healthcare Engineering*, *6*(1), 71–83. https://doi.org/10.1260/2040-2295.6.1.71

Reyniers, T., Deliens, L., Pasman, H. R., Morin, L., Addington-Hall, J., Frova, L., Cardenas-Turanzas, M., Onwuteaka-Philipsen, B., Naylor, W., Ruiz-Ramos, M.,

Wilson, D. M., Loucka, M., Csikos, A., Rhee, Y. J., Teno, J., Cohen, J., & Houttekier, D. (2015). International variation in place of death of older people who died from dementia in 14 European and non-European countries. *Journal of the American Medical Directors Association, 16*(2), 165–171. https://doi.org/10.1016/j.jamda.2014.11.003

Robinson, H., MacDonald, B. A., Kerse, N. M., & Broadbent, E. (2013). The psychosocial effects of a companion robot: A randomized controlled trial. *Journal of the American Medical Directors Association, 14*(9), 661–667.

Rockwood, K., Mitnitski, A., Richard, M., Kurth, M., Kesslak, P., & Abushakra, S. (2015). Neuropsychiatric symptom clusters targeted for treatment at earlier versus later stages of dementia. *International Journal of Geriatric Psychiatry, 30*(4), 357–367. https://doi.org/10.1002/gps.4136

Scerri, A., Sammut, R., & Scerri, C. (2021). Formal caregivers' perceptions and experiences of using pet robots for persons living with dementia in long-term care: A meta-ethnography. *Journal of Advanced Nursing, 77*(1), 83–97. https://doi.org/10.1111/jan.14581

Smith, G. E. (2013). Everyday technologies across the continuum of dementia care. *Annual international conference of the IEEE engineering in medicine and biology society. Annual international conference, 2013* (pp. 7040–7043). https://doi.org/10.1109/EMBC.2013.6611179

Torkamani, M., McDonald, L., Saez Aguayo, I., Kanios, C., Katsanou, M. N., Madeley, L., Limousin, P. D., Lees, A. J., Haritou, M., Jahanshahi, M., & ALADDIN Collaborative Group. (2014). A randomized controlled pilot study to evaluate a technology platform for the assisted living of people with dementia and their carers. *Journal of Alzheimer's Disease, 41*(2), 515–523. https://doi.org/10.3233/JAD-132156

Tyack, C., Camic, P. M., Heron, M. J., & Hulbert, S. (2017). Viewing art on a tablet computer: A well-being intervention for people with dementia and their caregivers. *Journal of Applied Gerontology, 36*(7), 864–894. https://doi.org/10.1177/0733464815617287

Van Patten, R., Keller, A. V., Maye, J. E., Jeste, D. V., Depp, C., Riek, L. D., & Twamley, E. W. (2020). Home-based cognitively assistive robots: Maximizing cognitive functioning and maintaining independence in older adults without dementia. *Clinical Interventions in Aging, 15*, 1129–1139. https://doi.org/10.2147/CIA.S253236

Wang, R. H., Sudhama, A., Begum, M., Huq, R., & Mihailidis, A. (2017). Robots to assist daily activities: Views of older adults with Alzheimer's disease and their caregivers. *International Psychogeriatrics, 29*(1), 67–79. https://doi.org/10.1017/S1041610216001435

WHO (2012). Dementia: A public health priority. *World Health Organization.* www.who.int/mental_health/publications/dementia_report_2012/en/

WHO (2020). The top 10 causes of death. *World Health Organization.* Geneva, Switzerland. www.who.int/news-room/fact-sheets/detail/the-top-10-causes-of-death

Wimo, A., Jönsson, L., Gustavsson, A., McDaid, D., Ersek, K., Georges, J., Gulácsi, L., Karpati, K., Kenigsberg, P., & Valtonen, H. (2011). The economic impact of dementia in Europe in 2008-cost estimates from the Eurocode project. *International Journal of Geriatric Psychiatry, 26*(8), 825–832. https://doi.org/10.1002/gps.2610

5   Aging in the Smart Home

Valerie Steeves and Jessica Percy-Campbell

Over the past decade, tech giants like Google and Amazon have brought a series of digital home assistants (DHAs) to market. These voice-activated devices, such as Google Home and Amazon Echo, enable users to easily access information, play music, make lists, and shop through a voice-activated interface with the Internet. They are also increasingly being marketed as resources that can help older people live independently. For example, a CNET review suggests that DHAs can help older parents and grandparents age at home by providing "help around the house", "hours of entertainment", and an easy way to "stay connected with loved ones" (Mitroff, 2019). Nurse Next Door Home Care Services adds that DHAs can also provide virtual companionship:

> Ask your Google Home to sing you a song or play one from the old days. Ask it to play a trivia game with you, or to tell you a story. Ask it questions like you would a real person. In a way, it's like having a digital companion as it learns the user's preferences and habits. For a senior who lives alone, a friendly voice available 24/7 can be a comforting option.

These devices ensnare older adults in a web of economic relationships that can have surprising results. This occurs because assisted living devices do more than providing support or care; they generate rich streams of behavioural and other data about their users and then transfer those data over the Internet to the corporations who designed the devices. These data are collected by these corporations precisely because they can be used to both predict and steer individual users' behaviour in ways that allow those corporations to generate profit.[1] From this perspective, DHAs targeting older adults are part of the emerging model of surveillance capitalism that "claims human experience as free raw material for hidden commercial practices of extraction, prediction and sales" (Zuboff, 2019, preface).

Accordingly, it is imperative that researchers begin to interrogate how this corporate practice reshapes the experiences of aging. As a first step in this direction, we focus on two common DHAs, Google Home and Amazon Echo, that are advertised as beneficial tools for older adults who wish to live

DOI: 10.4324/9781032617282-6

independently. The goal is not to conduct in-depth research of their capabilities, but to initiate a conversation about the consequences of using corporately controlled surveillance devices to provide care, possibly even replacing human caregivers. We begin by exploring the stated benefits of the two DHAs, by conducting a scan of popular older adult care and tech review websites that recommend their use. We then compare these benefits with the informational practices at the heart of these devices, as set out in corporate terms of use and other policies. That sets the stage to ask a number of interesting questions about how the flow of data is used to open the homes of older adults to commerce and to insert older adults into the networked marketplace. To acquire the data necessary to begin to answer those questions, we make some ethnographic observations about the advertisements that we were served online after we set up a Google Home account as an 80-year-old woman. We conclude by providing some preliminary recommendations and briefly outlining a research agenda to deepen our understanding of how surveillance capitalism mobilizes networked devices to reshape aging for commercial purposes.

DHAs and Assisted Living Devices

DHAs are just one part of a burgeoning industry in assisted living technologies targeting older adults in need of care. Schultz et al. (2015) suggest that this new industry is emerging because of a number of converging factors. First and foremost, as the baby boom generation has reached 65, the number of older adults in the population as a whole and the costs of caring for them have both grown exponentially. This shift in population patterns and budgetary demands has occurred just as the number of consumer electronics and networked communication devices in the marketplace has exploded. Government agencies under fiscal pressure are looking for ways to manage the costs of care for older adults, and technology companies looking to expand their markets have been happy to develop devices to meet older adults' needs. The result has been a proliferation of consumer products that are held out as supportive, cost-effective interventions that enable older adults to live independently and enjoy a better quality of life (Czaja & Lee, 2007).

The full extent to which assisted living devices can improve older adults' well-being is yet to be seen (Morris et al., 2013; Robillard & Hoey, 2018). The study published by O'Brien and colleagues (2020) is illustrative of these trends. It positions itself as the first attempt to research "the real-world use of voice-controlled intelligent personal assistants among older adults" (p. 176), and to do so, it analyses 125 consumer reviews posted on Amazon.com. Although the authors acknowledge that there are limitations to this approach – most notably that the reviews are both a weak proxy for the "actual utility" of using the Amazon Echo to care for older adults and a very small and non-representative sample of the opinions of older purchasers as a whole (p. 179) – they conclude that the device provides older adults with entertainment, companionship, reminders, control over the home, and easy access to emergency contacts.

They then call for further research to "encourage usage" and to help corporations improve device design (p. 179). Most notably, for our purposes, they fail to unpack the commercial nature of the reviews themselves. Although they acknowledge that "the purpose of these reviews was to provide opinions to other possible shoppers of Amazon Echo", the commercial nature of the testimonials is taken for granted. As a result, Amazon's role in curating the reviews, and the performative incentives that shape the actions of persons who write online reviews (including incentives to exaggerate the benefits of a product) (Shimp et al., 2007) remain unproblematized.

The growing body of critical qualitative scholarship that exists examining the experiences of older persons with these types of devices (Mortenson, Sixsmith & Beringer, 2016; Percy Campbell, 2023; Zwijsen et al., 2011) suggests that the data flows that these devices enable have negatively impacted older adults' experience of privacy and autonomy. Concerns have been raised, for example, that these technologies have

> the potential to be intrusive, subjecting residents to the gaze of others and making them feel watched . . . indirectly leading to changes in behaviour by being observed, or directly as a response to information and feedback as well as encouragement and interventions by the technology and/or service providers.
>
> (Mortenson, Sixsmith, & Woolrych, 2016, p. 111)

Particular attention has been paid to the "clinical gaze" (Mortenson, Sixsmith, & Woolrych, 2016, p. 111), and the ways in which information that flows to healthcare providers and family members may constrain the older adult's experience of the home as a place for retreat and ease.

Although we share those concerns, we seek to broaden the discussion by focusing on the corporate gaze and the commercial agenda that drives the information flows that are enabled by the technology. As a first step in this direction, we conducted a scan of popular older adult care and tech review websites to provide a window into how DHAs are positioned in the marketplace.

The Benefits of Aging in the Smart Home

We initiated our scan in 2020 by conducting multiple Google searches with key phrases such as "Google Home for seniors", "Amazon Echo for seniors", "Alexa for seniors", and "smart homes for seniors". We then read through the top 15 Google results for each search term, rejected duplicate articles or irrelevant results, resulting in a total of 47 articles with an average word count of 1,681. From here, we scanned the most frequently accessed blogs and websites[2] for a more careful analysis. The content we read enthusiastically (and often uncritically) endorsed both devices as tools that can help older adults age in place. However, closer analysis indicates that the stated benefits were largely to be enjoyed not by older users but by cash-strapped government agencies, children of older adults and the corporations that create and maintain the devices.

For example, although the discussion suggested that DHAs enable older adults to live independently, independence was framed as the solution to keeping the costs of care low because aging at home avoids the higher costs of being placed in a facility. Articles such as "Smart Homes for Seniors – Technology for Independent Living" (Paras, 2020) point to smart speakers as one solution to the high cost and limited availability of senior care: "Smart home technology is quickly proving itself as an affordable, user-friendly solution that has the potential to help the elderly grow old (on their own) in the comfort of their own home". Many located the real benefits of smart technology in the ability of care workers to keep a watchful eye from a distance through Amazon's "Drop In" feature (e.g., Pfender, 2018; Kane, n.d.). The implied gains in efficiency are largely located in the ability to monitor for negative outcomes such as loneliness, mobility problems and ineffective health monitoring without having to be with the older person. Since the technology is purportedly able to "care" for older adults and keep them "safe" in this way, costlier solutions such as live-in care or older adult care homes can be avoided.

This position clearly aligns with the managerial approach of government agencies that are seeking to lower public costs of caring for aging baby boomers (Schultz et al., 2015). The British Columbian government, for example, decreased funding for senior homes by 30% between 2001 and 2015 (Strauss & Xu, 2018), just as the baby boom generation approached their 60s. In this environment, technology becomes a win–win because it keeps older adults "safe" in a cost-effective way and aligns with their interests in avoiding the precarity of in-care facilities which are either privatized or staffed by poorly paid part-time workers (Strauss & Xu, 2018). This logic may be magnified in a post-COVID environment, given how crowding in long-term care facilities correlated with a high mortality rate among older adults during the 2020 pandemic (Payne, 2020).[3]

Similar to the ways in which surveillance systems for children are marketed, these devices are also framed with an emphasis on safety and peace of mind for the family members who are charged with providing care (see Marx & Steeves, 2010). For example, voice-activated devices are advertised as tools to help older adults with vision loss, poor mobility, or low finger dexterity that can make operating a smartphone difficult. They can also be helpful for those who need help reading small words on a screen, turning off the lights, locking the doors, creating hands-free shopping lists, or online shopping (Clark, 2017). In keeping with studies that have shown voice assistants to be helpful to dementia patients by "providing an ever-present voice that can answer the same questions again and again without losing patience and offer encouragement when needed" (Hoy, 2018, p. 86; Clark, 2017), family members are promised relief from the burdens of care, while still being able to "drop in" on their older relatives by watching them through Amazon Echo webcam or speaking to them through the speaker to give them a sense of comfort and familiarity (Pfender, 2018).

Concerns about loneliness are also alleviated by claims that voice-activated assistants can serve as companions through back-and-forth conversations. Although loneliness is considered to be the main difficulty that older adults experience (Perlman, 2004, p. 181), DHAs are held out as alleviating the need to visit in person, and care is accordingly restructured as a form of surveillance. For example, DHAs can monitor daily medications and be set to remind users to take their medication and avoid double dosing by responding "yes" or "no", when forgetful users ask "Alexa, did I take my medication today?" (Senior Living, n.d.). Checking in is replaced by the ability of older adults to quickly contact family in the event of an emergency through voice command via skills such as "Ask My Buddy" (Matthews, 2018). And children of parents with dementia are sometimes encouraged to routinely monitor user search logs to keep tabs on how their family member is interacting with his or her device (Clark, 2017).

While all of the articles in our scan presented an unwavering optimism about the possibilities of DHAs for older adults, only 14 of the 47 articles mentioned privacy. None mentioned the privacy concerns associated with the corporate collection of the data that DHAs harvest on an ongoing basis. Further, in one blog written for older adults and their caregivers, *Let's Say Thanks*, the author explicitly dismissed the possibility of an Alexa hack and encouraged older adults to "keep their privacy settings open" in order to experience the best results from Alexa's personalized services (Matthews, 2018). All three strategies – neglecting to talk about data privacy in any serious way, limiting concerns to individual perpetrators, and encouraging users not to use settings to restrict the flow of data – are at the least consistent with the fact that 14 out of the 47 articles are owned by marketing affiliates with direct ties to Amazon or Google.[4]

Market to Home: Operation and Terms of Use

Both Google Home and Amazon Echo have been highly successful in the marketplace: as of January 2019, over 52 million Google Home devices (Kinsella, 2018) and 100 million Amazon Echo devices (Bohn, 2019) had been sold worldwide.[5] In their most basic form, the devices consist of a smart speaker that is programmed to identify and respond to commands that are spoken after a user says a "wake word" (e.g., "Hey Google" or "Alexa"). In order to be able to respond upon request, the device is always listening for the wake word, unless the microphone is manually muted or the device is unplugged. Data is accordingly collected on an ongoing basis, and the flow of that data is governed by Google's and Amazon's terms of use statements and privacy policies, respectively. In this section, we provide a brief overview of the terms of those policies and the potential implications for older users.

Google Home

Like Amazon, Google operates on a notice and consent terms of service model whereby users, when they install the device in their home, tap "agree" to the terms on an associated app on their smartphone. Notice and consent models are meant to inform users of the types of data collection they are signing up for so that they may choose to "consent" to these practices in order to use the services. These types of consent-based policies are what allow data uses like Online Behavioural Advertising (OBA) to occur with permission from the user; rather than receiving contextual ads based on an individual search, ads follow users around the web based on their overall profile, which has been compiled based on data about the users' behaviour, location, and perceived interests (Barocas & Nissenbaum, 2009). It's important to note that if someone else, such as a friend or relative, sets up their smart speaker, the primary user of the device technically never "consented" to any form of data collection as someone else has gone through the process of "accepting" the terms for them.

The benefit of Google Home, from the corporation's perspective, is that the conversational data it collects can be used to finely tune each individual's profile; Google's advertising and other data services are accordingly more attractive to those who purchase them. Therefore, to maximize what it can collect from each user, Google Home can record and save all ambient noise captured by the device as a matter of course.[6] This includes quick questions directed to the device about the weather or the latest news, but it also includes other conversations and noises the device can hear when it is ostensibly "listening" for the wake word. The latter data is stored locally on the device itself. However, once a user speaks a wake word, the device both records the conversation and transmits the recording of the conversation (and any background noises) to Google over the Internet (Sarkar, 2019). That data is analysed remotely and a machine-generated response is transmitted back to the device which then plays it for the user.[7]

In addition, unless users change this setting, Google saves all conversational data, search history and location data indefinitely unless the user manually deletes it from the My Activity section of their profile (www.myactivity.google.com). Location data is requested when the user first initializes the system and, during the setup process, is asked to provide their home address. If the home address is not given, Google will glean location data from the IP address the device uses to connect to WIFI when it sends its data to Google (Data Security & Privacy, 2019). This enables Google to tag all the data it collects with an accurate estimate of where the user is physically located.

Data is also collected when users set alarms or timers or sync their device to their personal Gmail accounts or calendars so that they may receive reminders about their upcoming schedule. Similarly, data is collected when the device entertains users by streaming music connected through Spotify or YouTube Music. Additionally, the device supports third-party applications referred to as "Actions" (what Amazon calls "Skills") which generate rich streams of data that are then collected by Google. For example, WebMD is an Action that might be of particular interest to older adults with health issues. By saying "OK Google, talk to WebMD" or "Ask WebMD about the symptoms of dementia", users can engage directly with WebMD's online voice-activated service. Other examples of Actions include Headspace, an app for mental health and guided meditation, or Sun Life, which allows users to check their insurance balance and locate healthcare providers in the area. Memory Aid is an Action that can be utilized to remind users of anything they choose such as the keycode for their alarm system (Google Assistant, 2019). Google collects all search terms, video activity, engagement with ads, audio information through voice services, purchasing patterns, contacts, user-activity on third-party sites, and browsing history (Privacy & Terms, 2019).

The terms of use agreements that the user consents to upon installation then allow Google and its partner affiliates to use this data to "build better services" (Privacy & Terms, 2020). Google's privacy policy states it does not share users' personal information without consent:

> We'll share personal information outside of Google when we have your consent. For example, if you use Google Home to make a reservation through a booking service, we'll get your permission before sharing your name or phone number with the restaurant. We'll ask for your explicit consent to share any sensitive personal information.

In some cases, Google transcribes recorded conversations for third-party service providers but does generally not share recorded audio with them (Data Security & Privacy, 2019).

Further, although Google does not share personally identifiable information (PII) with advertisers except upon user request,[8] data collection is used to show users relevant ads and to "keep services free" (Data Security & Privacy, 2019). Ad selection is based on user profiles that are enriched by the data collected by the device. This data is particularly rich if users keep the default settings, as most do (Molla, 2018). Although Google shows personalized ads based on perceived interest, it also claims not to show ads "based on sensitive categories such as race, religion, sexual orientation or health" (Privacy & Terms, 2020). However, although this likely prohibits Google from collecting explicit health data (e.g., from an email or scheduled doctor's appointment), they may continue to target ads based on searches for health-related queries in certain jurisdictions; in that context, the queries themselves can be proxies for actual health conditions (Advertising Policies Help, n.d.).

Amazon Echo

While many Amazon devices such as Echo Show include a visual interface, due to space consideration, this chapter is limited to the traditional Amazon Echo model: a voice-activated speaker that does not include a camera or screen. Like other DHAs on the market, users can ask questions to Alexa, the personified voice-activated assistant which answers search queries using Bing.

Similar to Google Home, any time a user interacts with the device by either saying the wake word or touching the mic button, the interaction is recorded and sent to Amazon over the Internet, where it is analysed so a machine-generated response can be sent back to the device. Unless the user deletes the recordings through the Alexa app or on Amazon's website, they are saved in the cloud. Although the terms of use indicate that the Echo only records after hearing the wake word, there have been instances where background conversations have been recorded and sent to third parties and Florida police have (unsuccessfully) attempted to subpoena Alexa's recordings in a murder investigation (Copeman, 2020).

In addition to conversational data collected after the device recognizes the wake word, the Echo collects information when the device plays audio content on Amazon Music, Spotify or Pandora or performs other simple tasks such as making a to-do list, setting alarms, or telling jokes. Metadata is also collected when a user makes a phone call or sends a text to one of their contacts via voice command. Alexa-enabled products also create "voice profiles" so that they may automatically recognize and personalize engagement with specific users (Alexa Terms of Use, 2018). Accordingly, people who visit the house (and have not consented to the terms of use) may be profiled in this way.

Amazon also remembers online shopping preferences and uses them to serve targeted ads. Users can limit this by changing their "Advertising Preferences" on their user accounts (Help & Customer Service, n.d.). However, even if users take the extra step to opt out of personalized ads, the company states that they will still receive personalized product recommendations as well as ads on Amazon-affiliated sites (Amazon Advertising Preferences, 2019). Alexa will also sometimes incorporate paid promotions into its answers. For example, if you ask Alexa about buying toothpaste, you may get a suggestion to purchase Colgate (Estes, 2018a).

As Amazon is primarily a shopping-centric platform, Amazon Echo specializes in voice purchasing. Amazon Prime members can use their default shipping and payment settings to order online items through Alexa. For example, users in some US cities can order groceries from Whole Foods and receive delivery within two hours through Prime Now (Help and Customer Service, n.d.). Amazon also has its own set of unique Skills. For example, users with permission can use the "Drop In" Skill to remotely connect to another's device for a voice chat where a connection would automatically be made between devices without the receiver needing to accept the call (Help and Customer Service, n.d.). Another example is the Medication Reminder Skill which asks users to describe which medications they are taking by pill size and colour throughout the day.[9] Anyone can build their own Skill and add it to the Skill library for other users to try, although Amazon assumes no liability for these third-party services (Alexa Terms of Use, 2018).

Home to Market: A Snapshot of DHAs as Surveillance Capitalism Devices

As noted earlier, none of the corporate policies or the various blogs and articles discussing the advantages of smart home devices for older adults mention anything about how companies like Google and Amazon make profit. Under what Zuboff (2019) calls surveillance capitalism, both companies collect and commodify behavioural data; one of the primary purposes of doing this is to target ads back to users across devices. While Google monitors its users wherever they go online to feed its ever-expanding advertising network, Amazon seeks to keep users on its platform by making online shopping ever more efficient, personalized, and accessible (Pridmore & Mols, 2020). More recently, an experiment by a team of computer scientists has demonstrated that Amazon also profiles Alexa users for advertising purposes, despite Amazon representatives previously denying such practices in the media (Iqbal et al., 2022). Still, there is some crossover between the two competitors. Although online shopping is Amazon's main profit driver, the company is also the third biggest digital advertiser in the United States and is "veering closer" towards the kind of surveillance capitalism exemplified by Google (Zuboff, 2019). Likewise, Google Home offers voice-activated shopping through stores such as Costco by linking to Google Express. Regardless, whether the underlying goal is to enhance the experience of online shopping or the accuracy of behavioural ads, each relies on the ongoing surveillance of users and the collection and manipulation of the data that that surveillance generates.

This section explores some of the ways that embedding surveillance-driven commerce directly into the home might prove problematic for older adults. In the spring of 2019, we conducted a short experiment by setting up a Google account for a fictitious 80-year-old woman and, for the next three months, routinely searched for terms such as "dementia symptoms", "senior residences", or "how to be a good grandma" using both Google Home Mini and Google search. We then searched "news" and selected a few of the top 10 results and clicked through various news articles on random unrelated topics. We then screenshotted all of the Google ads that were shown on websites, at the top of search results, and in Gmail, when we browsed the Internet or used email under that user profile.

It quickly became apparent that our 80-year-old persona was being subjected to a minefield of problematic ads that followed her around the web. We received a plethora of ads for beauty products for older women, such as "flattering hairstyles for women over 50" or "how to make skin firmer" ads for beauty cream, and frequent requests to join older adults dating sites (e.g., SilverSingles).[10] The latter typically asked us to complete a long personality quiz and, upon completion, indicated that we would have to pay hundreds of dollars to sign up (which involves providing identifying information) to access responses behind a paywall. We also received many "investment opportunities", ads for multi-level marketing schemes or offers for 49.9% interest car loans and were repeatedly subjected to an ad for a non-refundable personal alarm system which has been reported as dysfunctional by a majority of reviewers.[11]

Of course, the practice of bad actors advertising online is not unique to Google. Bing, the search engine connected to the Amazon Echo, also has problems with fraudulent advertisements: recently, ads promoting tech support scams resulted in the suspension of 200,000 Bing advertising accounts (Garg & Hagelin, 2019). However, even though consumer-fraud-related risks are present for Internet users of all ages, some vulnerable members of older populations can be especially susceptible to risk as a result of lower levels of digital literacy, declining cognitive function or age-related conditions such as dementia (Mears et al., 2016).

This is particularly problematic for the older adults with health concerns. Although Google's own terms and service claims not to personalize ads based on health (Privacy & Terms, 2019), we found that any searches we did about health conditions, such as "dementia", were followed by a plethora of ads that followed our fictional older woman around the web on unrelated websites via associated devices. For example, over the course of two months, we consistently received ads for pills that claimed to enhance cognitive functioning, as well as ads for Alzheimer "quizzes" on unrelated websites. Clicking through the "quiz" once resulted in receiving even more ads for similar pills. This is particularly worrisome, since the FTC has issued warnings about the dangers of the types of fraudulent cognitive enhancement supplements which are promoted online (Small, 2019).

The prevalence of the $3.2 billion brain health supplement industry is a cogent example of how behavioural advertising can harm older adults. Following an investigation by *The Times UK*, Google has been recently scrutinized for profiting from ad space sold to companies who market fake memory improvement pills online (Bridge & Lay, 2019). These types of "pseudo-medicines" are not scientifically proven as there is no known cure or treatment for Alzheimer's (Hellmuth et al., 2019). In some cases, the supplements have been known to contribute to higher risks of stroke or even death (*ibid*). Although Google claims to have stopped selling ad space to these companies after *The Times* story was published (Bridge & Lay, 2019), it appears that these practices persist in some capacity.

Moreover, in 2014, the Privacy Commissioner of Canada (OPC) issued a report based on a complaint about Google Adsense targeting users based on sensitive medical information obtained through search. The OPC found that by following users around the web based on their behavioural data related to health, such as sleep apnoea, Google was in violation of s. 4.3 ("knowledge and consent needed to collect, use, and disclose personal information") and s. 4.36 of Schedule One ("express consent needed for the collection of sensitive information") of *The Personal Information Protection and Electronic Documents Act*. The OPC held that while "implied" or "opt-out consent" is adequate for non-sensitive information, "meaningful consent" is needed to deliver behavioural ads based on sensitive information such as health status (OPC, 2014). Following the report, Google agreed to fix this issue by disallowing advertisers to follow users based on health issues in Canada.

However, older adults exposed to behavioural advertising through their use of DHAs are already navigating hazardous waters. While Google promises not to share personal information with third parties, they fail to mention that information need not be personally identifiable in order to profile, target, and manipulate users. Online companies can still profile individuals without the need for their personally identifiable information (Bennett & Parsons, 2013). Fraudsters looking to sell faulty goods or services will often target older adults online. It follows that DHAs will only exacerbate this problem by linking the increasingly accurate profiles generated with data collected by DHAs with advertisers seeking to mobilize behavioural data for their own purposes who can deepen their messages by reinserting them into the home across an older user's devices.

Further, while making online shopping easier through voice command might be an attractive option for an older adult who has difficulty with a keyboard, it can also contribute to a new set of problems. Amazon Echo has voice-enabled shopping enabled by default, opening up the possibility that a person with poor memory might accidentally order the same item, or the wrong item, multiple times in a row. This is added to the concern that malicious actors could potentially seek to take advantage of this feature by ordering items through someone else's account without their knowledge (Hoy, 2018).

Security concerns simply add to the problem. Zhang et al. (2018) have shown that "skill squatting attacks" are a possibility with Amazon smart speakers. This is where malicious actors can publish fake Amazon skills which masquerade as other popular skills with names that sound similar. For example, if a user were to say "Alexa, open my Capital One skill", they may be redirected to a fake skill called "Capital Won" that exposes them to a phishing scam. Further, Barnes (2017) has shown that older Echo models are easily hacked through a physical vulnerability that may grant attackers remote access to the smart speaker. This allows a hacker to listen to the user's live audio without their knowledge. Depending on user settings, the fact that all interactions with these devices may be stored indefinitely is a recipe for disaster. As older adults are encouraged to use DHAs to keep track of their health issues, all it would take is a weak or duplicate account password for hackers to access troves of sensitive information. What's more, this type of health-related data collected in a commercial context is not protected in the same way it is in a medical institution, particularly in the United States, where medical information voluntarily stored on smart devices outside a hospital is explicitly exempt from the protections offered by the Health Insurance Portability and Accountability Act (HIPAA) (Lipman, 2016). And, as stated earlier, Amazon claims that it has no liability for breaches when a user takes advantage of any of its 60,000 third-party Skills, many of which are health-related (Kinsella, 2018).

It is also important to note that the notice and consent model working in these contexts has been designed to facilitate commerce (Steeves, 2016). The relatively weak protections it includes are typically rendered ineffective because most people do not read privacy policies to begin with, and the threshold of "opt-out" or "implied" consent for non-sensitive data collection for targeting is quite low (Lipman, 2016). In the case of Google Home and Amazon Echo, one person may set up the device for the rest of the household or, in the case of an older person living alone, the user's adult child or grandchild may set up the device for the primary user. This means that people whose conversations are captured by the devices are then subject to terms and conditions they have not ever had the chance to see (Percy Campbell, 2023). For example, anyone who poses questions to Google Assistant or Alexa may not be aware that whoever set it up will have access to those recordings through their account history. Further, those who had their device configured by someone else might not realize that their interactions are stored indefinitely, or that their data is being used to determine the types of ads they see online. They may not have even been presented with the possibility of opting out. While the use of notice and consent models for digital services is already weak to begin with (Barocas & Nissenbaum, 2009), it is even less effective in the context of the Internet of Things devices (Bracy, 2013) like DHAs.

There are some quick fixes that would be a move in the right direction. As Andrejevic notes, given an "unconstrained choice", most individuals would prefer not share their personal information with advertisers and third parties (2012, p. 86). For this reason, companies like Google and Amazon should make default privacy settings for smart home devices as restrictive as possible and at the very least require opt-in consent to use data for surveillance capitalist purposes, especially when older adults are using and such devices for caregiving functions.

Finally, just as consent is an important component of privacy, so too is the ability to retreat. In 1959, Erving Goffman presented the idea of the societal back stage, a space where individuals can relax as their true selves beyond the gaze of prying eyes and the need to perform (Goffman, 1959). Surveillance technology has chipped away at the "back stage" over the last couple decades, with smart homes being the most prominent recent example. Through the promise of an increased efficiency in performing everyday interactions, Google and Amazon have found ways to set up active microphones in the back stages of older adults' lives. This ability to monitor behaviour in the home impedes on the right to retreat as these devices constantly listen, always ready to record a person's latest thoughts expressed through search questions. As is the case with regular Internet browsing, the contents of those interactions are then saved, analysed and manipulated to serve the needs of corporate interests whose "imperatives are not necessarily our own" (Andrejevic, 2013, p. 189).

For those requiring assisted care, this process can be even more invasive. Relatives of older adults are encouraged to further infiltrate the backstage by "dropping in" unexpectedly through smart speaker cameras or with automatic audio connections facilitated by Amazon to make sure their loved one is "safe". They are also sometimes advised to monitor logged search interactions without the user's knowledge or consent. In short, older adults can suffer a loss of dignity when their privacy is invaded and that sense of invasion can be exacerbated when surveillance technologies are used to supplement or replace human care (Carver & Mackinnon, 2020). As a result, in spite of their lauded benefits of increasing autonomy and independence for the aging, DHAs may have the adverse effect of eroding dignity.

Conclusion: A Call for More Ethical DHAs and Further Research

To summarize, while Google Home and Amazon Echo are closely matched in functionality and their business models differ slightly, our preliminary analysis suggests that both work to entrench surveillance capitalism through the platformization of the home as a source of data. While Murakami Wood and Monahan (2019) recognize the significance of surveillance capitalism as the key driver in tech business today, they maintain that it is but one potential avenue of the platform economy. That is, rather than an increasingly rationalized world based on algorithmically generated predictions and suggestions, platforms that seek to monetize routine interactions of everyday life through disruptive new services may very well be the way of the future. Therefore, while surveillance capitalism might be the most prevalent business model right now, it is not inevitable or unchangeable (Murakami Wood & Monahan, 2019). This realization can help us think about the ways in which smart home services can be enhanced without the need for surveillance-based business models that work to benefit an already intrusive big data industry. The following conclusion explores preliminary recommendations to mitigate potential harms associated with Internet of Things technologies like DHAs.

Two top sellers of smart speakers, Google and Amazon, created notice and consent models that enable these devices to collect and store extensive behavioural data. While some settings can be changed to limit this, research has shown that most users do not change their default browser settings or device settings and that many users do not fully understand data collection and sharing practices (Molla, 2018; Lau et al., 2018). If these devices are to be used as care tools for aging in place, it is all the more important for tech companies to adequately protect user interests by default. For example, in order to access a smart speaker account, two-factor authentication should be mandatory as opposed to optional. Strong randomized account passwords should be forced by default and changed frequently. Moreover, privacy settings should be embedded into Alexa's back-and-forth audio interactions, as opposed to buried in the app settings on a linked smartphone, to allow Alexa or Google Assistant to periodically prompt users to delete their recordings and check up on their privacy settings via voice control (Lau et al., 2018).

Policy changes that diminish the reliance on notice and consent-based models would be a step in the right direction to limit harm caused by privacy intrusion, especially when many tech leaders argue that behavioural data collection should always be opt-in, rather than opt-out (Johnson, 2019). This would shift the burden of data protection responsibility away from the user. In turn, it could also help protect users with lower levels of technological literacy. Alternative DHA models that do not fall prey to the call of surveillance capitalism should begin to emerge as serious competitors to Google and Amazon. These devices should further embrace privacy by design and make strong security a key feature. User behavioural profiles should not be created without an opt-in function or true meaningful consent based on choice. The way that Duck Duck Go's search engine operates is a good example. The search engine does not track users, and ads are strictly contextual rather than behavioural. A more attractive DHA platform would include a similar model that does not track users or require their personally identifiable information, but that also charges a monthly subscription fee in exchange for delivering no ads at all. Moreover, third-party apps should be closely monitored by the parent company which should be held liable for abuse or misuse of data.

Finally, as privacy impact assessments are often too narrow to adequately predict other types of harm, surveillance impact assessments (SIA) and other ethical considerations should be conducted and made open to the public before new devices are released. These assessments should be updated often as capabilities and environments change (Bennett & Bayley, 2016). The rollout of Mycroft AI, an open-source and privacy-friendly DHA, was a step in the right direction (Pridmore & Mols, 2020). It demonstrates that alternative privacy-centric DHA models are in demand and that their development can be crowdfunded (Cardinal, 2019). Hopefully, the next few years will bring an influx of other DHA competitors to the marketplace as well.

The third and final recommendation includes a call for increased levels of public awareness. Security research has shown that current DHAs on the market are ripe with vulnerabilities (Hoy, 2018; Barnes, 2017; Zhang et al., 2018). This is concerning as malicious actors have an active interest in obtaining personal information including health status, location data and financial information. Lau et al. (2018, p. 2) found that smart speaker users of all ages may be unaware of privacy concerns associated with their devices:

> Smart speaker users, on the other hand, express few privacy concerns, but we find that their rationalizations exhibit an incomplete understanding of privacy risks, such as believing that they are 'not interesting' or that it would not be feasible for companies to comprehensively collect and store audio content.

As such, further efforts towards public awareness are required. While the tech media outlets such as *The Verge* or *Wired* do a decent job at critiquing security issues with smart home technology, they serve a niche audience. Websites geared towards older adults' wellbeing could stand to be more critical or balanced in their discussion of these devices. The unwavering tech enthusiasm noted in our media analysis is most likely to be convincing to families who either do not have the time to take care of their older adult family members themselves or have limited resources to put their loved ones into a care facility. This type of media supports a deceptive narrative by refusing to critically evaluate the possible negative repercussions of DHAs. This outcome is compounded by the fact that many assisted living blogs that recommend Alexa for older adults are actually Amazon advertising affiliates. Further transparency and public awareness campaigns are needed on this front.

General risk assessments aimed at public consumption are key for shifting the narrative. Media stories that sensationalize accidental data breaches are important for increasing awareness as they catch reader attention and make headlines. For example, we might recall the story about Alexa sending a personal conversation to a user's co-worker (Warren, 2018). However, those types of stories might seem like freak accidents or glitches. Instead, coordinated media campaigns dedicated to educating the general public on the potential *routine* risks involved in smart home systems for older adults could be beneficial. Momentum created by the recent rollout of the European Union's General Data Protection Regulation as well as backlash following the Cambridge Analytica scandal should be used to make data protection a campaign issue wherever possible. Ideally, this would push tech developers to secure their systems prior to product deployment as well as encouraging alternative competition. Perhaps most importantly, it could signal to policymakers the need to limit the acceptable use and data storage capacity of these devices.

Finally, qualitative studies that focus on how older adults actually use these devices for aging in place would be beneficial for further assessing privacy and surveillance risks. In addition, the link between smart speakers and targeted advertisements on associated devices has been understudied. If older adults are to use Google and Amazon smart speakers beyond their original intended uses, that is, as care tools for aging in place, we should be able to adequately assess how these behaviour patterns play into online profiling for advertisements or nudges towards online shopping. Finally, more extensive research on the types of advertisements older adults receive across the web in general help us understand both what types of companies are targeting older adults online, and how smart speaker use might feed into these profiles and potentially exacerbate negative outcomes. Overall, before commercial smart speakers can be celebrated as care tools in Canada, we suggest that further research on the privacy and surveillance implications of their usage by older adults is needed.

Notes

1 For example Alexa can steer conversations by responding to a command with follow-up questions designed to initiate 'give-and-take conversations with the voice assistant' (Priest, 2020).
2 There are also entire websites devoted to a particular device such as Alexa For Seniors (alexaforseniors.net).
3 The COVID-19 pandemic was also mobilized in marketing DHAs to seniors. For example, one article entitled "6 reasons to buy a Google Home for your

grandparents" (Mitroff, 2019) was retitled "6 Ways Seniors Can Use Google Home to Make the COVID-19 Quarantine Easier" and republished verbatim with the addition of a new introductory paragraph (Mitroff & Price, 2020).

4 These authors receive a commission from purchase links for Amazon Echo. For example, the sidebar of Senior Safety Advice says: "SeniorSafetyAdvice.com is a participant in the Amazon Services LLC Associates Program, an affiliate advertising program designed to provide a means for sites to earn advertising fees by advertising and linking to Amazon.com. As an Amazon Associate, I earn from qualifying purchases".

5 Depending on the model, the devices sell for between $50 (Echo Dot) to $150 (Echo Plus) on Amazon.com and $80 (Google Home Mini) to $400 dollars (Google Home Max) on Google's online store.

6 Until recently, this was the default setting for Google Home. At the time of publication, it remains the default setting for Amazon's Alex.

7 Google and Amazon have come under scrutiny for not disclosing the fact that the recordings may also be reviewed by actual humans, and for encouraging users not to opt-out of this feature as it will impact their quality of services (Crist, 2019).

8 Although it does share non-PII with "partners – such as publishers, advertisers, developers or rights holders".

9 For a demo of this Medication Reminder Skill, see www.youtube.com/watch?v=wmOcXAkloAg

10 It is important to note that SilverSingles has been flagged as a scam by many previous users. For reviews see www.sitejabber.com/reviews/silversingles.com

11 For Safesound personal alarm system reviews, see: www.highya.com/safesound-personal-alarm-reviews

References

Advertising Policies Help. (n.d.). *Support. Google.Com.* https://support.google.com/adspolicy/answer/176031?hl=en

Alexa Terms of Use. (2018). *Amazon.* www.amazon.com/gp/help/customer/display.html?nodeId=201809740

Alexa Terms of Use. (2020). *Amazon.* www.amazon.com/gp/help/customer/display.html?nodeId=201809740

Amazon Advertising Preferences. (2019). *Amazon.* www.amazon.com/adprefs/ref=hp_468496_advertisingpref2

Andrejevic, M. (2012). Exploitation in the data mine. In C. Fuchs, K. Boersma, A. Albrechtslund, & M. Sandoval (Eds.), *Internet and surveillance: The challenges of web 2.0 and social media* (pp 71–88). Routledge.

Andrejevic, M. (2013). Alienation's returns. In In C. Fuchs & M. Sandoval (Eds.), *Critique, social media and the information society* (pp. 191–202). Routledge.

Barnes, M. (2017, August). Alexa are you listening? *MWR Labs Publications.* https://labs.mwrinfosecurity.com/blog/alexa-are-you-listening

Barocas, S., & Nissenbaum, H. (2009, October). On notice: The trouble with notice and consent. *Proceedings of the engaging data forum: The first international forum on the application and management of personal electronic information.* https://ssrn.com/abstract=2567409

Bennett, J., C., & Bayley, R. M. (2016). Privacy protection in the era of "big data": Regulatory challenges and social assessments. In B. Van der Sloot, D. Broeders, & E. Schrijvers (Eds.), *Exploring the boundaries of big data* (pp. 205–227). The Netherlands scientific council for government policy. Amsterdam University Press.

Bennett, J. C., & Parsons, C. (2013). Privacy and surveillance. In *The Oxford handbook of internet studies* (pp. 486–508). Oxford University Press.

Bohn, D. (2019, January). Amazon says 100 million Alexa devices can be sold. What's next? *The Verge.* www.theverge.com/2019/1/4/18168565/amazon-alexa-devices-how-many-sold-number-100-million-dave-limp

Bracy, J. (2013, November). Are notice and consent possible with the internet of things? *International association of privacy professionals.* https://iapp.org/news/a/is-notice-and-consent-possible-with-the-internet-of-things/

Bridge, M., & Lay, K. (2019, March). Google cashes in on dementia pills that give patients false hope. *The Times.* www.thetimes.co.uk/article/google-cashes-in-on-dementia-pills-that-give-patients-false-hope-3gkqkll9v

Cardinal, D. (2019, January). Mycroft II provides voice-assist with data privacy. *Extreme Tech.* www.extremetech.com/electronics/283615-ces-2019-mycroft-ii-provides-voice-assist-with-data-privacy

Carver, L. F., & Mackinnon, D. (2020). Health applications of gerontechnology, privacy, and surveillance: A scoping review. *Surveillance & Society, 18*(2), 216–230.

Clark, J. (2017, May). Using the Amazon Echo to improve the lives of Alzheimer's patients. *Medium.* https://medium.com/@JaysThoughts/using-the-amazon-echo-to-improve-the-lives-of-alzheimers-patients-f5727560a5eb

Copeman, A. (2020, May 5). Is Alexa listening to me? *Tech Advisor.* www.techadvisor.co.uk/news/digital-home/is-alexa-listening-me-3785378/

Crist, R. (2019, July 13). Amazon and Google are listening to your voice recordings. Here's what we know about that. *cnet.com.* www.cnet.com/how-to/amazon-and-google-are-listening-to-your-voice-recordings-heres-what-we-know/

Czaja, S. J., & Lee, C. C. (2007). The impact of aging on access to technology. *Universal Access in the Information Society, 5*, 341–349.

Data Security & Privacy on Google Home. (2019). *Google Home help.* https://support.google.com/googlehome/answer/7072285?hl=en-CA

Estes, A. C. (2018a, February). Yes your Amazon Echo is an ad machine. *Gizmodo.* https://gizmodo.com/yes-your-amazon-echo-is-an-ad-machine-1821712916

Garg, N., & Hagelin, B. (2019). Ad quality year in review 2018. *Microsoft Advertising Blog.* https://about.ads.microsoft.com/en-ca/blog/post/march-2019/ad-quality-year-in-review-2018

Goffman, E. (1059). *The presentation of self in everyday life.* Anchor Books.

Google Assistant. (2019). *What it can do.* https://assistant.google.com/explore/c/6/

Hellmuth, J., Rabinovici, G. D., & Miller, B. L. (2019). The rise of pseudomedicine for dementia and brain Health. *Journal of the American Medical Association, 321*(6), 543–544. https://doi.org/10.1001/jama.2018.21560

Help & Customer Service. (n.d.). *Place orders with Alexa.* www.amazon.com/gp/help/customer/display.html?nodeId=201807210

Hoy, B. M. (2018). Alexa, Siri, Cortana, and more: An introduction to voice assistants. *Medical Reference Services Quarterly, 37*(1), 81–88. https://doi.org/10.1080/02763869.2018.1404391

Iqbal, U., Bahrami, P. N., Trimananda, R., Cui, H., Gamero-Garrido, A., Dubois, D., Choffnes, D., Markopoulou, A., Roesner, F., & Shafiq, Z. (2022). Your echos are heard: Tracking, profiling, and ad targeting in the Amazon smart speaker ecosystem. *arXiv preprint arXiv:2204.10920.*

Johnson, E. (2019, May). We should opt into data tracking, not out of it, says DuckDuckGo CEO Gabe Weinberg. *Vox.* www.vox.com/recode/2019/5/27/18639284/

duckduckgo-gabe-weinberg-do-not-track-privacy-legislation-kara-swisher-decode-podcast-interview

Kane, E. (n.d.) Echo show drop in skill for the elderly. *Senior Safety Advice*. https://seniorsafetyadvice.com/echo-show-drop-in-skill-for-the-elderly/

Kinsella, B. (2018, December). RBC analyst says 52 million Google Home devices sold to date and generating $3.4 billion in 2018 revenue. *Voicebot.ai*. https://voicebot.ai/2018/12/24/rbc-analyst-says-52-million-google-home-devices-sold-to-date-and-generating-3-4-billion-in-2018-revenue/

Kinsella, B. (2019, January 2). Amazon Alexa skill counts rise rapidly in the U.S., U.K., Germany, France, Japan, Canada, and Australia. *VoiceBot.ai*. https://voicebot.ai/2019/01/02/amazon-alexa-skill-counts-rise-rapidly-in-the-u-s-u-k-germany-france-japan-canada-and-australia/

Lau, J., Zimmerman, B., & Schaub, F. (2018). Alexa, are you listening? Privacy perceptions, concerns and privacy-seeking behaviors with smart speakers. *Proceedings of the Association for Computing Machinery on Human-Computer Interaction, 2*, 1–31. https://doi.org/10.1145/3274371.

Lipman, R. (2016). Online privacy and the invisible market for our data. *Penn State Law Review, 120*(3), 777.

Marx, G., & Steeves, V. (2010). From the beginning: Children as subjects and agents of surveillance. *Surveillance & Society, 7*(3/4), 192–230. https://doi.org/10.24908/ss.v7i3/4.4152.

Matthews, I. (2018, May). Alexa for seniors, get yourself a personal assistant. *Let's Say Thanks*. www.letssaythanks.com/alexa-for-seniors/

Mears, D. P., Kuch, J. J., Lindsey, A. M., Siennick, S. E., Pesta, G. B., Greenwald, M. A., & Blomberg, T. G. (2016). Juvenile court and contemporary diversion: helpful, harmful, or both? *Criminology & Public Policy, 15*(3), 953–981. https://doi.org/10.1111/1745-9133.12223

Mitroff, S. (2019, February 23). 6 reasons to get a Google Home for your grandparent: An elderly relative in your life can benefit from a smart speaker. *cnet.com*. www.cnet.com/how-to/buy-google-home-for-your-grandparents/

Mitroff, S., & Price, M. (2020, March 28). 6 Ways seniors can use Google Home to make the COVID-19 quarantine easier. *cnet.com*. www.cnet.com/how-to/6-ways-seniors-can-use-google-home-to-make-the-covid-19-quarantine-easier/

Molla, R. (2018, May). Google's privacy changes are mostly marketing. *Vox*. https://www.vox.com/recode/2019/5/9/18537250/google-privacy-tracking-cookies

Morris, M. E., Adair, B., Miller, K., Ozanne, E., Hampson, R., Pearce, A. J., Santamaria, N., Viegans, L., Long, M., & Said, C. M. (2013). Smart-home technologies to assist older people to live well at home. *Journal of Aging Science, 1*(1), 1–9.

Mortenson, W., Sixsmith, A., & Woolrych, R. (2016). The power(s) of observation: Theoretical perspectives on surveillance technologies and older people. *Ageing and Society, 35*(3), 512–530. https://doi.org/10.1017/S0144686X13000846

Murakami Wood, D., & Monahan, T. (2019). Editorial: Platform surveillance. *Surveillance & Society, 17*(1/2), 1–6. https://ojs.library.queensu.ca/index.php/surveillance-and-society/index | ISSN: 1477–7487

O'Brien, K., Liggett, A., Ramirez-Zohfeld, V., Sunkara, P., & Lindquist, L. A. (2020). Voice-controlled intelligent personal assistants to support aging in place. *Journal of the American Geriatric Society, 68*, 176–179. https://doi.org/10.1111/jgs.16217

OPC. (2014, June). Use of sensitive health information for ads raises privacy concerns. *Office of the privacy commissioner of Canada*. www.priv.gc.ca/en/opc-actions-and-decisions/investigations/investigations-into-businesses/2014/pipeda-2014-001/

Paras, C. (2020). Smart Homes for seniors – Technology for independent living. *DIY smart home solutions.* www.diysmarthomesolutions.com/smart-homes-for-seniors-technology-for-independent-living/

Payne, E. (2020, June 25). Crowding a key factor in high long-term care death rates, new research says. *Ottawa Citizen.* https://ottawacitizen.com/news/local-news/crowding-a-key-factor-in-high-long-term-care-death-rates-new-research-says

Percy Campbell, J. (2023). *Aging in place with Google and Amazon smart speakers: Privacy and surveillance implications for older adults* [Doctoral dissertation]. http://hdl.handle.net/1828/15095

Perlman, D. (2004). European and Canadian studies of loneliness among seniors. *Canadian Journal on Aging, 23*(2), 181–188.

Pfender, E. (2018, June). Amazon Echo instructions for seniors – What you need to know. *Caregiver Connection.* https://caregiverconnection.org/amazon-echo-for-seniors/#tab-con-8

Pridmore, J., & Mols, A. (2020). Personal choices and situated data: Privacy negotiations and the acceptance of household Intelligent Personal Assistants. *Big Data & Society, 7*(1), 1–13. https://doi.org/10.1177/2053951719891748

Priest, D. (2020, August 8). Alexa is starting to ask questions: How should we respond? www.cnet.com/news/alexa-is-starting-to-ask-questions-how-should-we-respond/

Privacy & Terms. (2019). *Google.* https://policies.google.com/privacy

Privacy & Terms. (2020). *Google.* https://policies.google.com/privacy

Robillard, J. M., & Hoey, J. (2018). Emotion and motivation in cognitive assistive technologies for dementia. *Journal of Aging Science, 1*(1), 1–9.

Sarkar, S. (2019, December 20). Is Google Home listening to me? *Tech Advisor.* www.techadvisor.co.uk/feature/digital-home/is-google-home-listening-me-3695908/

Schultz, W. L. (2015). A brief history of futures. *World Futures Review, 7*(4), 324–331. https://doi.org/10.1177/1946756715627646

Senior Living. (n.d.). Three reasons seniors need voice command devices. *Senior Living.* www.seniorliving.com/article/3-reasons-seniors-need-voice-command-devices

Shimp, T. A., Wood, S. L., & Smarandescu, L. (2007). Self-generated advertisements: Testimonials and the perils of consumer exaggeration. *Journal of Advertising Research, 47*(4), 453–461. https://doi.org/10.2501/S002184990707047X

Small, B. (2019, April). Ask a health professional before popping that pill. *Federal trade commission consumer information.* www.consumer.ftc.gov/blog/2019/04/ask-health-professional-popping-pill

Steeves, V. (2016.) Now you see me: Privacy, technology and autonomy in the digital age. In G. DiGiacomo (Ed.), *Current issues and controversies in human rights.* University of Toronto Press.

Strauss, K., & Xu, F. (2018). At the intersection of urban and care policy: The invisibility of eldercare workers in the global city. *Critical Sociology, 44*(7–8), 1163–1178.

Warren, T. (2018, May). Amazon explains how Alexa recorded a private conversation and sent it to another user. *The Verge.* www.theverge.com/2018/5/24/17391898/amazon-alexa-private-conversation-recording-explanation

Zhang, N., Mi, X., Feng, X., Wang, X., Tian, Y., & Qian, F. (2018). Understanding and mitigating the security risks of voice-controlled third-party skills on Amazon Alexa and Google Home. *Preprint, arXiv:1805.01525* [cs]. http://arxiv.org/abs/1805.01525

Zuboff, S. (2019). *The age of surveillance capitalism: The fight for a human future at the new frontier of power*. Public Affairs.

Zwijsen, S. A., Niemeijer, A. R., & Hertogh, C. M. (2011). Ethics of using assistive technology in the care for community-dwelling elderly people: An overview of the literature. *Aging & Mental Health*, 15(4), 419–427.

Conclusion and Future Directions

L.F. Carver

Hacking Your Age started with the thesis that aging is an intersectional experience which can be enhanced or threatened by biohacking, biotechnologies and/or gerontechnologies depending on who controls them and how they are used. Shared understandings of key terms, such as biohacking, biotechnology and gerontechnology, have been established and issues such as equity, access and practical usage, as well as the dangers of misuse explored. The influence of social determinants of health on access to these methods was discussed, especially for those who are low income or in developing countries without the medical infrastructure to support more complex forms of biohacking and biotechnology.

Worldviews and religions can introduce additional questions that deepen the radical life extension conversation. The already extended life expectancies in many countries have created a huge challenge as medical systems attempt to manage multi-morbidity. However, keeping older persons healthier for longer, and compressing the period of disease and frailty at the end of life, could help mitigate (rather than exacerbate) unequal (gendered) caring duties – because more older men would survive to help care for their aged parents. And yet, keeping people alive longer runs the risk of simply extending the period of time we can stave off death rather than actually improving our *quality of life* in late life. In the end, what really counts is adding life to years versus years to life.

Future Directions

For those who are lucky enough and can afford to make the choice, aging in place at home – where we know the best places to get groceries, the safe places to walk and who our neighbours are – is usually the first choice (Carver et al., 2018). To facilitate aging in place, the AgeTech industry (the intersection of digital innovation and longevity) is creating and marketing products designed to appeal to older adults and/or their caregivers.

Technology development aimed at older adults – AgeTech – has mostly focused on assistive devices, health-related devices and entertainment as well as robotic and bionic technology. Virtually all types of AgeTech include data recording with Wi-Fi-enabled transmission of personal data for purposes of

DOI: 10.4324/9781032617282-7

monitoring health and/or optimizing the technology (Misselhorn et al., 2013; Pedersen et al., 2018; Pike, 2019). And, as we have discussed throughout the book, this data is vulnerable to leakage, exploitation and re-purposing for off-label use such as advertising for consumer products and services, market research, inclusion in amalgamated mega-databases, and/or by criminal entities who intend to exploit it for profit (Mortenson et al., 2015).

Contrary to some stereotypes, older adults are embracing technology. At least two-thirds of Americans over 65, and 82% of Baby Boomers, use the Internet (Anderson & Perrin, 2017), and many own wearable devices such as smartwatches and/or fitness trackers as well as smartphones and tablets. Utilizing AgeTech to manage age-related deficits or functional challenges could be the key to aging in place and remaining independent. For example, radio-frequency identification (RFID) tags combine a tiny radio transponder, a radio receiver and a transmitter and can be placed under the skin. These RFIDs can be used to hold passwords, to open doors, turn on lights, and/or log into the computer (the self-implantation of RFIDs is a relatively common biohack). As a gerontechnology, for those older adults who have a loss of grip strength, the implantation of an RFID tag that opens the door could increase independence. For those with a loss of manual dexterity, having the RFID log into the phone or tablet could reduce social isolation by facilitating social connection through technology. RFIDs can also store personal information, for example, name and emergency contacts – and someday, maybe, will include GPS tracking and/or biosensors that could warn of impending heart attack or other traumatic health event.

An expanding AgeTech market is the use of devices for entertainment or to stave off loneliness. Touched on briefly in Chapter 4, social robots have been developed for entertainment, but are often suggested to older adults as a replacement for pets. These "robots" have artificial intelligence (AI) that is designed to interact with and provide comfort to the user.[1] Some of these are designed to simulate pet dogs and cats. They are not intended to fool the user into believing they are real, but rather to fill the void between visits from loved ones, or in the absence of a beloved dog or cat. Although most healthy older adults dismiss the idea of a robot toy as a pet, valuing the reciprocal relationship between living beings (Carver, 2022), they can, nonetheless, find social robots entertaining or amusing.

However, much like the digital home assistants (DHAs) discussed in the previous chapter, social robots (including robopets) collect data on the user's emotions and social patterns. An array of sensors that record facial expressions and conversations. And, these social robots are always "on" in order to respond when addressed or touched by the user (Misselhorn et al., 2013). Human user data is required in order to instruct the robot as to the "correct" response. Unless manually shut down, human activity is recorded everywhere the robot is – including the bathroom and bedroom. Emotional data – all those feelings that flicker across our faces through the day are recorded and sent to the cloud.

Since social robots have cameras and sensors on board – why not direct those away from the person/user and towards their environment? The existing technology built into social robots could be used to meet the challenges that a wide range of people experience – including older adults aging in place. Social robots could be created to warn a user *of any age* that someone is at the door, the kettle is boiling, or the smoke detector is shrieking, as well as providing more mundane services such as reminders for a video call or doctor's appointment. The GPS technology in "self-driving" cars could be uploaded into a robopet which would then provide navigational support to tourists or people with visual impairment. These existing technologies could be repurposed to enable people with some types of functional impairments to live independent lives. Further, using affordable items, such as robot pets, to support independence addresses many of the moral and ethical concerns linked to the greater access to life-enhancing/-extending biohacks and biotechnologies by the privileged raised throughout this book.

These technologies and others developed to support older adults and "combat" challenges of aging may put already vulnerable older adults at a greater risk of exploitation. We need to use the *buyer beware* adage because, for example, the same RFIDs that open doors and store passwords could open users to GPS tracking or information collection without their permission or even knowledge. As mentioned earlier, social robots can be entertaining for the user while siphoning information and sending it to a third party to exploit.

There are those who suggest the benefits that older adults get from being observed, especially the ability to age in place, outweigh the costs of being watched and overseen (Moffat, 2008). However, constant surveillance creates a paternalistic environment where older adults are being protected from themselves, which can be considered a violation of the right to independence and self-determination (Minuk, 2006; Percival & Hanson, 2006). Technology is evolving so quickly that governments can't keep up with its uses and misuses. At this time, the onus is on users to understand the risks and prevent misuse.

The longevity economy represents all economic activity linked to products and services for older adults and is an estimated $7.6 trillion annually.[2] It is to be hoped that if older adults direct their purchasing power to choose devices that support independence without infantilization, they can change the trajectory of this industry. When entertainment-type AI is reconfigured so that "toys" like robot pets function as smoke detectors, or as dash-mounted devices that warn of impending collisions, or as a guide to find the grocery store in a new town, these types of technologies can support independence, rather than amusement.

Conclusion

AgeTech can be utilized by both healthy and health-challenged adults to stay safely at home. At the present time, it often means living in a "watched world", with DHAs, cameras, and door sensors to monitor users (Carver & Mackinnon, 2020). Although the ubiquitous use of cameras and voice monitoring equipment in a home environment can raise privacy concerns, and impact human mental health (Yang et al., 2018), they can also be the key to independence.

Most of us would prefer to live longer, healthier lives. However, the use of biohacking, biotechnology, and gerontechnology to do so raises challenging and complex issues. The recurring theme in *Hacking Your Age* is that we must consider the moral and ethical questions, including privilege and access to life extension/enhancement. Of paramount importance is whether a few people should be allowed access to expensive life-extending technology, while a much larger number lack access to basic needs like clean water, safe housing, and economic stability.

Notes

1 https://theconversation.com/robopets-using-technology-to-monitor-older-adults-raises-privacy-concerns-132326
2 www.oxfordeconomics.com/recent-releases/the-longevity-economy

References

Anderson, M., & Perrin, A. (2017). Tech adoption climbs among older adults. *Pew Research Center*. www.pewinternet.org/2017/05/17/tech-adoption-climbs-among-older-adults/

Carver, L. F. (2022). Pandemic and pets: Attachment to non-human animals and well-being during the Covid 19 pandemic. *One Health Innovation*, *1*(1). https://ojs.library.queensu.ca/index.php/onehealthinnovation/article/view/16190/10575

Carver, L. F., Beamish, R., Phillips, S. P., & Villeneuve, M. (2018). A scoping review: Social participation as a cornerstone of successful aging in place among rural older adults. *Geriatrics*, *3*(4), 75–90. https://doi.org/10.3390/geriatrics3040075

Carver, L. F., & Mackinnon, D. (2020). Health applications of gerontechnology, privacy, and surveillance: A scoping review. *Surveillance & Society*, *18*(2), 216–230. https://ojs.library.queensu.ca/index.php/surveillance-and-society/index

Minuk, L. (2006). Why privacy still matters: The case against prophylactic video surveillance in for-profit long-term care homes. *Queen's Law Journal*, *32*(3), 224–277.

Misselhorn, C., Pompe, U., & Stapleton, M. (2013). Ethical considerations regarding the use of social robots in the fourth age. *GeroPsych: The Journal of Gerontopsychology and Geriatric Psychiatry*, *26*(2), 121–133. https://doi.org/10.1024/1662-9647/a000088

Moffat, P. (Ed.). (2008). Should we tag people with dementia? *International Journal of Palliative Nursing*, *14*(2), 56–56.

Mortenson, W., Sixsmith, A., & Woolrych, R. (2015). The power(s) of observation: Theoretical perspectives on surveillance technologies and older people. *Ageing and Society*, *35*(3), 512–530. https://doi.org/10.1017/S0144686X13000846

Pedersen, I., Reid, S., & Aspevig, K. (2018). Developing social robots for aging populations: A literature review of recent academic sources. *Sociology Compass*, *12*(6). https://doi.org/10.1111/soc4.12585

Percival, J., & Hanson, J. (2006). Big brother or brave new world? Telecare and its implications for older people's independence and social inclusion. *Critical Social Policy, 26*(4), 888–909.

Pike, G. (2019). Biometrics and robot dogs challenge Illinois Law (Legal issues). *Information Today, 36*(1), 26–27.

Yang, G., Yang, J., Sheng, W., & Li, S. (2018). Convolutional neural network-based embarrassing situation detection under camera for social robot in smart homes. *Sensors, 18*(5), 1530. https://doi.org/10.3390/s18051530

Index

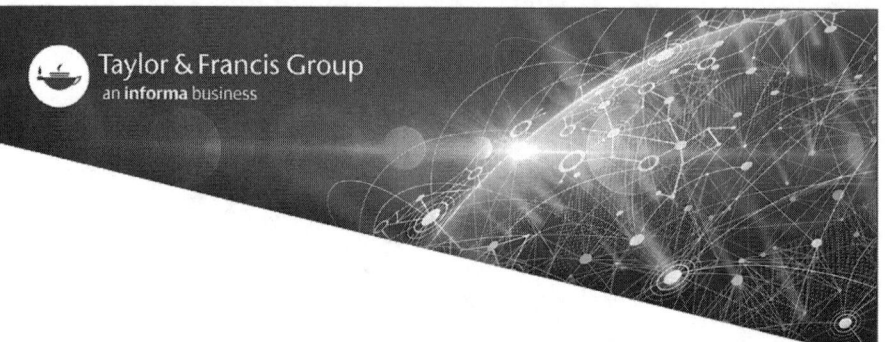
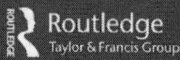
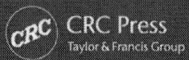